THE ADDICTION MONOLOGUES

THE STORY OF ADDICTION AS TOLD BY ADDICTION

RICHARD D. CAMPBELL

CONTENTS

A Dialogue - The Solution to Addiction

FOREWORD

In the pit of my stomach and throughout my limbs, I feel that there is something quite wrong. Not lining up. That square peg in a round hole kind of feeling. You know what I mean. The shift has taken place. I vigilantly look around to see if anyone has noticed the discrepancy.... I had misplaced my script.

Like a bird on a wire, feeling exposed and silhouetted against the gray sky, there is a disoriented feeling. Other birds come and go all around me. They are infrequent and without warning. Flitting to and fro.

These were familiar scenes of life for me. There was an exhausting and steady stream of keeping every thought straight. There were the kids, friends, and family. Then, one day, on a Tuesday morning in September, the bomb went off between my husband and I. This bomb contained a mixture of addiction and unfaithfulness. Devastating everything I thought to be typical. The time had come.

When my husband and I met Rich Campbell, we were already into the therapy scene with other counselors and had reached a point of ambiguity. I was ready to try something new and found Rich much by mistake. The person I thought we would meet with had a full schedule. Our second session with Rich was revealing. He asked if we wanted the traditional counseling or if we were up for a more imaginative style. It was clear from the start that this creative and fearless man understood clearly what others before him had not. Trauma. My husband and I led a life of carefully crafted coping skills. We had our way of life. Sure, our life was uncommon and most people would have told you we were a very fun couple to go to dinner with. The shift for us came when the alcohol would emerge from somewhere. It always found its way in. We found that in our trauma we practiced daily, it was like steady drips of water on a solid rock that eventually made a deep hole. This hole held the bomb.

As it turns out, continuing to meet with Rich over the next two years taught us things we did not realize we needed to embrace or knew was possible to possess. We learned how to articulate and guide our own questions back to our own beliefs and unhealthy systems we had set in place long ago.

"Not as an excuse, but an explanation" was a common phrase quoted by Rich that gave confidence and validity to our values and ponderings. If he believed we could get there, we started to believe it ourselves. That was six years ago.

Finding out that we can work our way to wholeness without living out our distinctive addictions was a welcome surprise to us. We found an uphill path out of the past trauma and daily hiding that was grueling and heartbreaking at times. As we continued to trust our own pain and learn to be okay with it, Rich would urge a bit more out of us for a journey to unity and healthy choices as a couple. It was time to find more than a current solution for the current addiction. The Addiction Monologue is a rare look into the sights, sounds, and smells of addiction that will open up some aha thoughts and cause you to stop and set the book down and ponder at times.

So like the solitary bird on a wire, sitting placidly taking in the scene, the sky clears, clouds flow behind steadily, he considers his next move, confidently looking at his surroundings; he spreads his wings and takes off.

Isn't it about time?
Julie Blakely

UNDERSTAND

What you are about to read is an unconventional perspective of an ugly topic in our culture, the topic of addiction. It's not only an ugly topic, it's an ugly epidemic. Think about all of the people you see in a day. Not just the ones you know, but ALL of them. See the faces. At least one of every four people you see each day are directly impacted by this ugly topic. It is my hope that if we look at this ugly topic from a different perspective, we will start to think differently about it, and about the people who are part of its story.

This is the story of Addiction,
as told by Addiction.

PREFACE

"All warfare is based on deception."
Sun Tzu, Art of War, 1:18

The inspiration for the Addiction Monologues come from my very eclectic set of experiences. From individuals as diverse as C.S. Lewis, the author of the Screwtape Letters, to Sun Tzu, who was Lewis's predecessor by some 2,600 years, many of which have examined the struggles humans face between each other as well as those faced from within. Both of these great writers, as well as many diverse experiences, have influenced my journey and perspectives.

During my career as an intelligence officer in the United States Air Force, I gained an appreciation for understanding the thought and decision making process of my potential enemies. If you understood the how and why of their thoughts, you would have insight to "predict" their future actions. It was during this time in the military that I was introduced to the writing of Sun Tzu, a Chinese military strategist, who lived in the sixth century BC and wrote the Art of War. He said,

> *"All warfare is based on deception. Hence, when able to attack, we must seem unable; when using our forces, we must seem inactive; when we are near, we must make the enemy believe we are far away; when far away, we must make him believe we are near. Hold out baits to entice the enemy. Feign disorder, and crush him. If he is secure at all points, be prepared for him. If he is in superior strength, evade him. If your opponent is of choleric temper, seek to irritate him. Pretend to be weak, that he may grow arrogant. If he is taking his ease, give him no rest. If his forces are united,*

separate them. Attack him where he is
unprepared, appear where you are not expected."
(1:18-24)

After I left the military, I began working with individuals who struggled with addiction. And it didn't take long to recognize the strange parallels that existed between my previous career and my work in the field of addiction treatment and recovery. I shifted from supporting the rescuing of American hostages, to seeking to understand how individuals could be taken hostage from within by addiction. In the latter situation, shooting the bad guy would not be an option. I began to wonder if Sun Tzu knew something about addiction because it too, like warfare, seemed to thrive upon the deception of self and others.

As I worked with individuals and their family's, I discovered metaphors and personifications helped them grasp the disease of addiction in new ways. Ways that helped them more effectively engage the treatment they needed to save their life or the life of a loved one. Addiction, as a destroyer of everything good, is easily seen as evil. If addiction was a person what would they be like? Charming? Smart? Attractive? From what I've seen, addiction would have an IQ of at least two thousand and appear charming and telepathic, all the while hating your guts and desiring to kill you. Addiction, the brain disease that hijacks the limbic system of our brain, cannot only read your thoughts, it can create them.

Everything you are about to read is based upon current addiction science and actual events in the lives of real people. The names and details of the events have been modified to protect confidentiality. Parts of the monologue are very ugly and will be difficult to read. People die. The purpose of the Addiction Monologues is to bring addiction to life in a new way. I want you to walk with me and view addiction from a very different perspective. Do you want to help someone struggling with addiction get into treatment? Are you thinking about becoming an addictions counselor? Would you like to better understand this plague on humankind? Whatever your motivation for reading, I hope what follows will challenge you to see the struggle of those facing addiction differently. I also hope it will lead you to view addiction from a whole new perspective. What does addiction value? How does it think? How does it make decisions? How does it take someone hostage from within? If we fail to learn and understand the answers to these and similar questions, we won't win this fight. Addiction is a brain disease unlike any other. It is also a disease of opportunity. And given the opportunity, it will take you to the grave.

The Addiction Monologues is written from the perspective and voice of addiction. Why call it a monologue? Because it is only about one voice. A dialogue is the discussion of multiple views with the goal of understanding and compromise. Addiction longs to hear only one voice – its own. Welcome to the addiction monologues.

PART 1

THE ADDICTION
MONOLOGUES

1

LET ME INTRODUCE MYSELF

I love situations like John's because they are so emotionally exhausting for you humans. No one is asking you to reveal your secret because no one knows you have a secret. The kicker is you're DYING to tell someone but you know you can't because the guilt and shame will overwhelm you. And that, my friend is the perfect pain to bring you to me. You see, I will take that pain away. I promise.

John believed me.

We were formally introduced when he was thirteen. I remember the burning feeling in his throat that first time. It was like fire. Once the physical discomfort passed, the warm feeling of sedation created by the alcohol as it absorbed into his blood stream quickly flowed over him. It was the first time he could remember not feeling the pain of the racing thoughts that never stopped. He had never told anyone about the pain of those thoughts because he simply couldn't put it into words. Intense emotional pain is like that. It was the start of a great relationship for me. John's young brain quickly surrendered control. In this same surrender, I took his mother several decades earlier, I wouldn't have expected anything less. I'll be sharing more about John later.

OK, here's my first secret I'm going to let you in on. You think it's about the alcohol. It's not. That's what makes it so easy for me to take humans — you think so one dimensionally. I am a god of many facets — like a fine cut diamond I reflect and amplify the light around me. I could have just as easily used the THC in marijuana or those prescription pain meds in the medicine cabinet to take John. But I give people choices, at least at first.

I am a mystery to most of you, even though in some way I've touched virtually every one of you. But you remain oblivious to my presence. Some don't believe I exist — even though I've been around as long as the human race. And those who do acknowledge my existence don't believe they will ever meet me, even though they see and talk to me every day. I am Addiction. And because I'm feeling generous, I'm going to share some of my story and deep secrets with you.

I am a brain disease. And as a brain disease, if you have one, a brain that is, you're fair game to me. There isn't a brain I can't hijack. I'm generally modest, but I have to say I'm unlike any other disease. If you didn't know, your brain has more mathematical complexity than your known universe. Within those five to six inches between your ears flows over one hundred neurotransmitter chemicals. Your one hundred billion neurons have some forty quadrillion possible wiring combinations. That's a lot of neurological real-estate to control. How do I do it? I go straight to the command center and take control of key portions of your limbic system and a couple of key neural pathways into your cortex. While I can influence a variety of areas of your brain, my objective is to take control of your fight or flight responses. This allows me to take first place in your life. I also get to drive. I am a great driver. You begin to see and perceive me in terms of your survival, as a matter of life and death. You come to believe, as you should, it is I who sustains you and without me you would die.

Some call me a "medical condition." I prefer disease as it sounds more powerful and fitting. I operate at all levels of human existence and interaction - biological, emotional, relational, and spiritual.

As a spiritual disease, I detach you from your values, your beliefs, your sense of purpose, and the truth. I'll help you to learn a new truth, my truth. When I take control, I'll have you attack your family and friends on our behalf. You'll help me isolate them, destroy your relationship with them and, if I'm lucky, you'll help me take them too. There is nothing more powerful, at least from my perspective, than the nasty degrading things you'll say and do to those you claim to love. Each one - you, your loved ones, your friends – will become a part of my masterpiece of devastation. I know I'm powerful, but I'm still amazed and impressed by the fact that I am invisible to you. To the untrained eye, I'm unseen and, for the most part, I like it that way. I may not always receive the public credit I'm due, but, for those I take, *in the end, in a wonderfully terrifying moment of clarity, they know it's me.*

Having said all this, I'm counting on you to keep my secrets. Besides, even if you do share what I'm about to tell you, no one will believe you. What follows is a truly great story. It's my story. The names of those who carry my story are not important to me, but they should be to you because you know them and see them every day. Some of them drove your kids to school this week, served your food today at lunch, made recommendations to you about your investments, and woke up next to you this morning. I hope you enjoy my story, I know I do, and, if I have my way, you'll soon be part of it.

2

FOREPLAY & CONCEPTION

Like many stories, mine begins with the journey to conception. My conception, however, is uniquely different within each human being. While an egg and sperm are the key ingredients for human conception, I can be conceived through a variety of events and circumstances.

The seeds for my birth come from your pain. It could be physical, emotional, or spiritual pain. It doesn't matter to me. I'm not particular about the source of your pain either. As long as it's strong enough to entice you to search for me, I'll make sure you find me. I know what you're thinking (and I'm not kidding when I say that), "Why would I search for you?" It's a valid question; you're thinking no one in their right mind would search for me. The fact is people aren't actually looking for me, they're looking for what I "promise" – relief from their pain – at least for the moment. You will do almost anything to stop feeling your pain.

Don't misunderstand what I'm saying, I'm definitely not stupid, and for the most part neither are you. Although there are always exceptions to how I operate, I'm generally not overt, unless I think it will work. Sometimes life works as my ally and sets everything in place. All I have to do is shout, "jump" and you leap into my arms like a small child shouting, "Catch me!" More often, however, there are many individuals and events that I take advantage of, as I score the soundtrack to capture your heart. It's really your brain I'm capturing but that sounds less romantic. Let me introduce you to some of my people.

JULIE

Julie's story is just one of millions. She's a confident and attractive young woman with long, jet-black hair. The air of confidence she gives off is reassuring to some, but off putting to others. She was raised in a small farming community in the Midwest. Her parents, Dan and Cindy, kept busy as the owners of the local IGA grocery store. From the outside the facades were idyllic. Hardly the place one would think of to be associated with pain. Hot summers, beautiful autumns, long cold winters with lots of snow. Her family lived just on the edge of town in a new housing development. They were at the end of a cul-de-sac. A corn field met the side of the yard. The house was a modern two-story with a nondescript lawn. They literally had a white picket fence around the brick house. A symbolic but completely ineffective form of protection.

Julie was the younger of two children. As a child, she loved to be the center of attention from the time she was a toddler. Growing up she was full of energy and always curious. By the age of five, the combination of her long, black hair, dark eyes, and engaging smile was mesmerizing. Julie was always close with her bother Adam, who was two years older. As small children, Julie was like his shadow, always following him and wanting to a part of whatever he was doing. When Adam was seven, he began Cub Scouts. Julie was heartbroken and couldn't understand why she wasn't allowed to go with him to his scouting events.

As a teen, her energy and desire for attention, combined with her slight, yet athletic physique, helped her to excel and become a star in the high school athletic programs. Volleyball, gymnastics, and track were her passion and took up much of her time, much to the dismay of her male classmates, who attempted to pursue her. Even with what many would consider to be stunning looks, she never seemed to be interested in boys or dating. She did however have your typical small circle of girl friends, most of which were also athletes.

Julie was seven when her journey to me began. She was confused about how the encounters with her uncle made her feel. Her mind at this young age was not developmentally ready to handle what was happening to her. The encounters with her uncle continued until she was thirteen. It was Adam that walked in on them by accident one day and discovered their, "secret." Julie actually defended her uncle out of a combination of her own guilt and confusion. In a unique negotiation with Adam, their uncle promised never to touch Julie again, and Adam promised not to reveal what he had discovered to their parents. As Julie's confusion and guilt grew in its intensity, so did her feelings of worthlessness. But it was more than a feeling, it was her belief.

PETER

A handsome, athletic young teen, he was the second of four children. His parents lived an average, middle-class existence – both worked to make ends meet. His brother Dan was almost four years older, and they never really connected as siblings. For that matter, he didn't connect with his other two siblings either. His sister, who was two years younger, kept to herself. His little brother Jake had downs-syndrome.

His years prior to becoming a teen would be considered by most to be uneventful. His parents had mild concerns that he was a bit lost as the middle child and wasn't connecting with the family or with many friends. As he entered middle school, he had the opportunity for his first big trip away from his family. He wasn't actually going anywhere alone – he was going on a middle school youth retreat sponsored by the church his family attended. Peter's expectations for the trip were high. His parents were excited over his enthusiasm and for the opportunity for him to connect and develop stronger friendships with kids his age. It was never clear to his parents what exactly happened on the youth group retreat. Peter came back different, but not in the way his parents were hoping.

All his parents could manage to piece together from him was that Peter had somehow been humiliated in front of his peers by one of the youth leaders. Anytime they tried to talk to him about the trip he would get angry. What his parents failed to recognized was the pain Peter was feeling. I recognized it. And I knew exactly what I was going to do with it. Family friends encouraged his parents by telling them that a little middle school razzing was no big deal, and Peter would eventually snap out it. I love it when you downplay the pain experienced by someone else. It's the best way I know to intensify the emotional pain felt deep within their heart. Fortunately for me, humans often fail to understand the intensity of emotional pain felt by someone else. The intensity of the pain is determined by them - the one experiencing it, not by those watching it.

Eventually Peter did "appear" to snap out of it. After all, for you it's all about appearances. The anger his parents had seen in his eyes just after the retreat was no longer visible. In reality, what was behind that anger was humiliation, but they didn't see that. The whole idea of "out of sight, out of mind" is a wonderful human myth I love to exploit. While the appearance of humiliation was not detectible to the casual observer, or even his parents, it was still very much present below the surface, deep within Peter's soul. Sort of like the black mold that continues to grow behind a freshly painted wall. With humans, it's only a short distance from humiliation to my favorite feeling of all, shame. I'm not sure if shame is a feeling or a belief in humans. Not that it matters. Feel it, believe it, I really don't care which you choose as long as the end result brings you to me. And Peter came running.

It was a crisp fall day, the first day you could see your breath. School had just gotten out and Peter was heading home. If you asked him now, he wouldn't even be able to tell you the names of the guys who asked him if he wanted to get high. It wasn't so much that he wanted to get high as he just wanted to stop feeling. The memory of what happened on that youth retreat didn't just haunt him, it hunted him. The story about being humiliated in front of his peers by a youth leader was a lie, the first of many. The first night of the retreat, one of the older male teens repeated his own "abuse" history, and sexually acted out with Peter as an unwilling, yet participating partner. This particular individual was a year ahead of Peter in school and hardly a day went by during the school year that Peter didn't come face to face with the memory of that night. The euphoric feeling of the delta-9-tetrahydrocannabinol, which you call "weed," clouded his mind. For the first time, he felt something akin to peace. It was so easy. Funnel some emotional noise toward a human for any length of time, and when it's removed, you call it peace. In reality, it's just quiet. Call it what you want. Just remember, I made it happen.

ANTON & SUSAN

Anton, by my standard, was a geek. Most of you would probably have a different first impression of him, but I knew his thoughts. From the outside he was tall, slender and slightly muscular in his physique. He grew up in the middle of four siblings as the classic middle child. He and his brothers spent their summers racing quads through the woods or kayaking on the river that ran through the vast property of his home. He grew up with every toy imaginable to a teenage boy; snow machines, dirt bikes, jet skies, and boats. They even had a two hundred foot zip-line from their professionally built treehouse. Everything had an appropriate place and was always cleaned after it was used. His world was as close to perfect as humanly possible. Perfect was defined, and controlled, by his parents.

He had a steady girlfriend through much of high school. It was just by chance they had met one day during one of the annual celebrations in the small community near where he lived. She attended a public school and was not part of his family's class structure - which at times made things awkward between them. While his parents never openly disapproved of his relationship with her, Anton did have his moments of doubt about her. Did she want to date him because of who he was on the inside, or just because of his family's money and the access to everything that came with it. That question wasn't just confined to his girlfriend. It was a thought filter Anton used with virtually all of his friendships.

After graduating from a private high school, he was accepted to a well respected mid-sized private university in the Midwest. Dad wanted him to study business finance, and dad always got what he wanted. Anton lived on campus for the experience of socializing and had actually done well in his classes. His relationship with his high school girlfriend ended within a month of starting school. His parents' divorce during his junior year of college caught him completely and utterly off guard. His almost perfect world had evaporated. Both of the extravagant homes he grew up in were sold and everything changed. The whole experience made him cautious about close relationships, or any relationship for that matter. He couldn't articulate the pain he felt, all he could feel was a mix of sadness, frustration, and anger. He would struggle between not knowing what he was feeling, not knowing how to express what he felt, and not wanting to feel anything at all. In spite of that, he managed to successfully complete his coursework and graduated as a software engineer.

He dated a handful of women during college but didn't make a real connection with any of them. Connection requires feelings, and feeling his emotions felt dangerous. He did, however, feel a greater sense of urgency to find a life partner after finishing college, while at the same time still feeling off balance with the break up of his parents marriage. I love unhealthy tension, don't you? He ended up seeking a serious relationship with Susan. They met in his senior seminar class the last semester at school. They ended up getting married a year later. Given the wealth of his family and the interest that could generate from the opposite sex, Anton's relationship choices had been relatively safe. The thought or belief that people were only interested in him as a means to his family's money and lifestyle kept him from truly connecting with anyone. Even himself.

Susan had grown up in Kansas City. Since money wasn't an issue, Anton took a position in Kansas City at a company called Image Tech, as a financial analyst in order to be close to Susan's family. He could have had a job in his father's flag ship business but was still angry at him over the divorce. Image Tech did have corporate affiliations with one of his father's companies, which may have been why he got the job, at least that's what I keep telling Anton. Susan's family came from a solid middle-class background, but the wealth of Anton's family was still way out of their league.

Anton and Susan purchased a home in a nice development and quickly settled into their social and work routines. Anton had done well in his new position and was securing a reputation beyond his father's last name and corporate connections. While they had planned to put off starting a family for several more years, they had become the proud parents of twin daughters just two years after moving to Kansas City.

Every birthday is special, but the twins third birthday would put Anton on a new path in life. He was twenty-eight at the time. Susan needed him to make a quick run to the local grocery for some last minute items for the birthday party. It was a trip he had made hundreds of times. It wouldn't take long. It was early summer, sunny and warm. The light was green. But something was different. Everything went into slow motion like a movie passing one frame at a time. The light was clearly green - but it just didn't make sense – why was that red car there – broadside – in front of him? The driver was looking straight ahead but Anton's eyes focused on the little girl sitting in the backseat. She looked about five years old and was sitting next to the window closest to him. Her blond, curly hair just touched her shoulders.

She was looking right at him and locked eyes with him. I remember him thinking to himself, what pretty eyes she...BOOOOOM! The panic was instantaneous. Anton couldn't breath or see anything. When he was six Anton's older brother would hold him down on the floor and put a pillow over Anton's face and torture him for what felt like an eternity without air. His faced burned, but it wasn't hot, it was like a carpet burn. Even though it felt like his brother holding him under the pillow he knew he hadn't been transported back in time twenty plus years. He still couldn't breathe which made the sense of panic worse. His head hurt, for that matter his whole body hurt. After what seemed like several minutes, which was actually only a few seconds, he was able to take a breath. His previous moment of visual bonding with the little blonde girl in the red car was interrupted by the sound of reality and the exploding airbags in his SUV. The young couple driving the car with their daughter in the back seat had driven through a red light. The couple sustained minor injuries and were kept overnight at a local hospital. Anton ended up with two black eyes, but not a scratch more. The girl who locked eyes with Anton was pronounced dead at the scene. The face of the young girl looking out the window in the last seconds of her life was forever imprinted into Anton's mind.

6
CONCEPTION

All of these stories have one thing in common. Each one is sacred to me. The combinations of emotional devastation, trauma, secrets, shame, and guilt are magical for me. They're part of my conception. The seeds of my conception are unique and they often go unnoticed. When they are noticed, someone close to the situation – usually a family member or friend - quickly moves to cover them over so they will be hidden – which is exactly what you want to do if you want seeds to grow. You call them secrets. I call them treasured moments – the moments of my conception.

Humans make a big deal about prenatal care. You take vitamins, attend special classes, and take strange ultra sound pictures where you point out all of your body parts. You read books about giving birth and raising children. You fix up special rooms and buy furniture, and you have parties anticipating the birth. Me, I don't need any of that. Ignore me – at least initially. Let me fester in your deep dark place of pain. Focus on your loneliness, the rejection, the feeling of being overlooked, drink in the pain.

Unlike you, my conception doesn't take place between your legs. I prefer the space between your ears. The womb that carries me is found deep within the one hundred billion neurons you call your brain. It starts in what you refer to as your heart. Not the muscle that beats in your chest, but rather that place deep within your being some describe as your soul. In a similar fashion to the wounding of the egg as it is pierced by the sperm at the moment of human conception, my impregnation occurs through the wounding of your soul. How this takes place is different for each person. For some, my impregnation leaves barely a scratch at best upon their soul, which then requires a complex combination of actions and reactions to result in my full-term birth. For others, my impregnation desecrates their soul and rips it into pieces too numerous to count.

7

JOHN

Remember John? I was conceived in John when he was six. He and his older brother lived in a comfortable middle-class family. His father had a successful law practice and his mother was active in church and the community. She filled photo albums with "family pictures" from vacations to exotic locations. The images were as far away in distance as they were from the reality of their home life. You see, I already had a relationship with John's mom.

My conception in John was at the hands of his babysitter and her boyfriend. It was during a time when John's dad was attempting to thwart my relationship with his wife and he had shipped her off to, "treatment." His older brother was allowed to fend for himself, but John needed a sitter to watch him during the evening hours. The sitter and her boyfriend began engaging in sexual acts with John on the very first night they watched him. They swore him to secrecy. I love children, but obviously not for the same reasons you do. It is so easy to manipulate the mind of a child. They'll believe anything, including whatever is happening to them is their fault, and if they tell it will be their fault even more. John's sexual encounters at his young age lit up portions of his brain that were not ready to be turned on yet, pun intended. He was confused about how it made him feel and why something that made him feel so good needed to be kept a secret – it didn't make sense to him – but those were the rules he was given. Rarely did a day go by that he didn't think about how his babysitter and her boyfriend made him feel, and all of the confusion that came with those feelings. Fortunately for me, John continued to live with the confusion in silence, frustration, and intense loneliness.

The confusion and guilt John felt as he moved into his early teens served me well. He wanted to tell his parents about what the sitter and her boyfriend had done to him, but when his first attempt brought only shame, guilt and a lot of yelling from his dad, he gave up on the idea of telling anyone. His dad was emotionally exhausted and angry at everything. My timing was perfect. Mom had just gotten back from, "treatment" about a month earlier and I had just renewed my relationship with her. She really missed me. It was great getting back together; John's dad was off the chart jealous of our relationship and he was taking it out on John and his older brother. The family was nicely wrapped up in my wonderful chaos – I think you call it hell – but I'm in control, so I get to call it what I want. I don't think they even knew John was alive. And that's exactly what I kept whispering to him.

He became aware of my support and how much I cared for him after one of his parent's arguments. Their arguments, which seemed to last for hours, included screaming profanities mixed with the sound of doors slamming. John hated it. The yelling was constant, but the unexpected slamming of the doors was like exploding RPG's on the battlefield. John had retreated to his room. It was a refuge from the chaos but at the same time a tomb. While he wanted to escape from the yelling, when it stopped, the silence in his room was deafening. He could feel his heart beating. It reminded him of the first night after being molested. He laid in his in bed that first night with nothing but his thoughts of what had happened and the sound of his heartbeat. The thoughts, memories, and emotions swirled endlessly in his mind creating a combination of confusion and pain he couldn't put words to – and even if he could, he didn't have anyone to tell. He had to do something. I was so proud of him. He wasn't alone in his room any longer. I was with him, as well as the bottle of vodka he had discovered in the garage and had brought to his room.

After our formal introduction around the age of thirteen, John and I developed a close and trusting relationship. He trusted me to take away his pain, and I did, as long as he did his part and kept me close. Trust is important to me. I expect it; I deserve it and demand it. Why shouldn't I? Who else is going save you from your pain? Humans are hardwired to withdraw or escape from anything that they believe is causing them pain, whether it's physical or emotional. The sources of physical pain are usually relatively easy for you to figure out. Emotional pain can be more complicated and mysterious. I like mysterious because it allows me to fill in the blanks for you. You have this false belief that if you could just know the "truth" behind your pain, it will magically go away. It doesn't exactly work that way, but I'm all about the truth…sort of, I don't actually take the pain way, I just make it so you don't feel it.

I kept John sedated and for the most part unaware of his pain. When he was a senior in high school he had managed to secure a part-time job working in the shipping department of a small printing company. He was a hard worker and did a good job. I was fine with that. My relationship with John was about striking a balance to provide for maximum duration of our time together. I had plans for him and his family. With some additional training and a couple of courses at a community college he eventually moved into a position as a graphic designer for the company. He liked the title "graphic designer," but we both knew he was mediocre at best. For the most part he kept his personal relationship with me separate from his work. But I eventually joined him at work as well. He put up a confident façade, but he lived in fear that someone would eventually discover his relationship with me and expose him for the fraud we both knew him to be.

Actually it's a little more complicated than that. I knew he was a fraud. All humans are frauds. The fears that ran deep within his soul, and also in yours, are often so deep that they are not visible on the surface. They are like deep ocean currents. You feel the subtle influence of them on the surface, but you're not consciously aware of them. It's a nagging sense that something isn't right, but you just can't put your finger on it, it's a mystery. What often results is transferred emotional or spiritual pain. The pain get's a label, but it's rarely correct. It really doesn't matter to me if it's labeled correctly or not. People see me as the solution. I solve their most pressing problem - pain.

John thought he was over the shame and guilt of what had happened to him. I kept my promise – I took that pain away. Technically, I just made it so he didn't feel it. But I was starting to get bored, it was time for something new. All that sedation was making him numb. He needed to feel something. But it would have to be something that would work well with the alcohol. I really hope you can appreciate the artistic nature of my work. It's all about placing just the right thing in front of you at just the right time. For John it was time to revisit all those feelings of sexuality. I love the internet.

John's discovery of pornography worked perfectly to awaken the reward pathway of his brain. You think I don't understand neurobiology - that's fine, you just keep thinking that way. The reality is I know it better than you do. The reward pathway is located near the top of your limbic system. That's the address where I live if you ever want to get in touch with me. So the alcohol sedated his grey matter above the reward pathway and the porn activated the pathway itself. It worked perfectly! Not only that, the more John engaged the porn to produce what he thought were real feelings, the more guilt and shame he felt, which then required greater amounts of alcohol. Tell me I'm not a genius.

John had been cycling between alcohol and porn for over a year when it happened. John's older brother and his wife had a crisis at their store one morning and asked John to stay with their daughter while they took care of things. John's ability to "hold" his alcohol was so good that his brother and sister-in-law had no clue I had him in an almost continual state of intoxication. His boundaries between the feelings generated by the porn and the feelings that erupted as his niece Julie crawled onto his lap were blurred. His hands began to dance in a playful game that triggered both excitement and shame in his mind, and confusion in Julie's. Uncle John eventually named it their, "secret dance" and told her that it had to be kept just for them. The grief and shame he felt after what began that morning, and continued until his "secret dance" with Julie was discovered by her older brother, sealed his relationship with me for life, his life.

8

KAREN

Karen is what you humans would call, "a full sized woman." I just call her Porky. Well obviously I didn't start with that nickname but once she was mine I could call her whatever I wanted. She began preparing for my birth around age twelve or thirteen. It wasn't a spectacular conception by any means; her parents just always seemed to be preoccupied with the crisis of the moment created by her older brother. In the midst of all the family chaos created by her brother, Karen remained quiet. She was quiet because she always had food in her mouth. It had become her comfort, and I'm not against comfort, especially when it's pseudo comfort. Pseudo comfort is what humans seek during my gestation. I like it because it doesn't actually address the source of your pain and it gives you a false confidence that you are actually doing something to make "it" better. In Karen's situation "it" was the feeling of being ignored by her family, the feeling of being overlooked, not important, insignificant. It's a dull pain at first, but thankfully for me, it would grow in intensity.

My birth in Karen wasn't a particularly hard labor, it just took longer, but that's the way I planned it. You know - the whole joy in the journey thing. I remember sitting on the couch with her cuddling under the blanket while she consumed massive quantities of theobromine, phenethylamine and caffeine. Her locus ceruleus would kick in and bathe her brain in dopamine and norepinephrine. For Karen it didn't get any better than this. It was truly love at first bite. For the non-chemists out there I'm talking about chocolate. It was her first stop, and one she would return to many times, on her relationship journey with food – her best, and come to think of it, only friend.

I sure hope you're beginning to see this. My superior understanding of your brain chemistry, emotional neediness, and spiritual emptiness, combined with your total ignorance of the same, allows me to move the game pieces on the board in such a fashion that your coming to me is a given. This isn't about if we'll meet, it's about when. And that of course will be at the time and place of my choosing. As a medium, food isn't the most glamorous, but it's ubiquitous, there's no human fear associated with it, and your society accepts it. It's a relatively easy medium for me to use, even boring at times, but it works, and I find that I can build upon it to create some really great works of art - my art! I like to think of myself as a brain surgeon, artist, psychologist, pastor, priest, super model, lover, and savior all combined. You humans are touchy about the ~ g – o – d ~ word so I'm not going to openly claim it, but we all know the truth. But I've digressed, back to porky Karen.

By age fifteen, Karen's weight had surpassed two hundred pounds. Her feelings of being overlooked and insignificant felt five times that heavy. Eating had become like breathing for Karen. The dopamine and serotonin released from eating chocolate would calm her anxiety and make her "feel" loved. When she wasn't shooting – I mean eating chocolate, she was doing a combination of carbohydrates, proteins and fats that produced a narcotic like sedation that would cover over the emotional pain of rejection. Who needs cocaine when you can get saccharin at every corner gas station and grocery store? Sometimes subtle is more powerful than audacious.

Once conceived, I don't need much. I feed off your neglect, not neglect of me, you don't even know I'm there resting within your mind. I'm talking about how you neglect your pain. You pretend, both to yourself and others that your pain doesn't exist. It's the learning curve of denial. You begin by denying your pain, and later after my birth, you deny my presence. But let's not get ahead of ourselves on your pain – there will be plenty of time for that later.

Karen's pain came from a sense of abandonment by her family, and everyone else for that matter. From your "technical" perspective, Karen's attempt to "soothe" this pain through eating created a behavioral pattern that ultimately resulted in the construction of a neurological path. As her eating continued, the neurological path was strengthened by the growth and wiring together of her neurons, or brain cells. Eventually, in a magic moment that only I know, a shift occurs, a transfer of power and control takes place inside the brain. Happy birthday to me, happy birthday to me, come on! Sing with me!

You seem really uptight. You know I think I could help you. Have you ever tried delta-9-tetrahydrocannabinol?

9

BIRTH

My birth usually goes unnoticed which is fine by me. I usually don't make my public appearance until I know my position is secure. For humans, birth is pretty hard to miss. Labor pains begin and follow a pattern of increasing intensity and frequency, culminating in your birth. My birth takes place deep inside your mind in your limbic system. Most of you can look at your birth documentation and know the exact date and time of your birth. You will never know the exact time of my birth - that's only for me to know.

10
JULIE

Adam, Julie's older brother, had turned sixteen just a few months earlier. He and his parents were enjoying the freedom his driver's license provided for them, especially when he needed to be at his part-time job at a local coffee shop early on Saturday mornings. This Saturday, however, someone had screwed up the schedule and Adam ended up finishing his shift early. He made plans with a couple of his friends to hook up at the skate park and was going to swing by the house to pick up his skateboard. As he turned the corner onto their street he could see his uncle's truck was in the driveway.

Julie had just started volleyball that year and had a skill training clinic that Saturday at school. Dad had to be at the store, and mom was out of town visiting one of her crazy sisters. With Adam having to work on Saturdays, his dad had arranged for his brother John to chauffeur Julie to the training clinic that morning.

Julie's heart was pounding. Her encounters with her uncle had moved to a new level of intensity over the past year. Things had changed. Julie had started to menstruate a few months earlier and the new intensity of her hormones was overwhelming and made any rational thought difficult. Feelings of fear, confusion, and excitement alternated with every beat of her heart. Her mind raced – I shouldn't be doing this – I can't believe I'm doing this – could I get pregnant – I'm not supposed to like this – we shouldn't be here – did I just hear a car door slam? That last thought was lost in the haze of the moment.

Adam came in through the garage and headed upstairs to his room to get his skateboard. In the back of his mind he was expecting to see his uncle, either in the kitchen or more likely in the living room watching TV, but he didn't appear to be in the house. He liked his uncle. Prior to getting his license he frequently took Adam and his sister for regular outings to the movies, the mall, or fishing. As he rounded the corner at the top of the stairs and headed down the hallway time slowed down. It felt like a scene from a movie. His ears

31

picked up a sound that didn't fit. It was out of place. It was coming from his sister's room. The momentary confusion made him wrinkle his forehead; she's supposed to be at that volleyball thing she was whining about last night, Uncle John was going to take her. Why is his truck here but he's not – who is here? His heart began to pound. John had left the bedroom door open just enough to provide some privacy but still let them hear if someone had come into the house, which was obviously an untested theory as it had clearly not worked. Adam's eyes focused through the open space of the not quite closed bedroom door. His heart was pounding, but I think he stopped breathing.

What John had originally called their secret dance had progressed far beyond the fondling that started some seven years earlier. While every muscle in Adam's body seemed to freeze, he somehow managed to make sound come out of his mouth as he pushed open his sister's door. Can you say awkward? I think even I was embarrassed. For John and Julie it was guilt and shame. For Adam it was anger and confusion. For me it felt like Christmas and a birthday party all wrapped into one.

While Julie's mind had been racing to make sense of what was happening between her and her uncle, every thought in her head seemed to crash against her skull as if an emergency brake had been pulled on a high speed train. She knew her encounters with her uncle were moving beyond her comfort level, but they had never come even close to getting caught. She immediately started to blame herself for the two of them being in her bedroom. If she hadn't forgotten her permission slip for the volleyball clinic that morning, they wouldn't have come back to the house. Actually, that wasn't true, but I wasn't going to tell her. John had the missing permission slip in his pocket the whole time. He had picked it up off of the kitchen table when he came into the house that morning to take her to school. Julie didn't remember she needed it. I think we were just about to the school when I suggested to John that we could create an opportunity to spend some alone time with Julie, hence his decision to forget he had the permission slip in his pocket. He thoughtfully stayed for a few minutes in the parking lot just to make sure Julie was all set, secretly hoping they would send her home to get the slip. It all worked perfectly and as soon as they walked back into the house to look for the paperwork, I suggested to John that they start their search in Julie's bedroom.

I had to work fast after Adam stumbled into her room to make sure I didn't lose any ground, and if possible could grab some more. I used Julie's shame and confusion to get her to beg Adam not to tell their parents, because after all it was partially her fault (as I had been telling her all along) and if something is your fault you get punished, like not being able to play volleyball, which was the only thing giving her any sense of value. The limbic system of John's brain went into full protection mode and began to build multiple justification schemes to protect me. It made me feel warm all over. Adam was making a lot of sound but nothing coherent. All of this went on for several minutes until I moved John to gain control of the situation and start the negotiations to insure my safety.

I immediately suggested he try either a minimization or misunderstanding strategy. John quickly went with the story line that what Adam had walked in on was a first time event that began in complete innocence. To John's surprise - and relief - Julie followed his lead and backed up his story. Both continued to dispute the reality of what Adam thought he saw. In the end it was agreed upon by all that what happened between John and Julie shouldn't have happened, that it would never happen again, and it would not be in anyone's best interest to tell Julie and Adam's parents. In the end, even if John's extracurricular activities with Julie had been exposed to her parents, I still could have used the events of that day to my ultimate end game. However, the chosen option did create more secrets, and if you haven't figured it out, I love secrets.

PETER

Just when spring was about to arrive, life offered me another great opportunity in Peter's life. I still remember the day. It was bright and sunny and the last traces of snow were melting away. Peter had overslept that morning, probably because he didn't actually start sleeping until about 3:30 that morning. I liked staying up late and secretly talking with him. His oversleeping put the family bathroom schedule off track, which led to an exchange of endearing family pet names between Peter and his younger sister - fatso, loser, porky, pot boy! After they had used them once or twice they would recycle them with the addition of some profane modifier to increase the effectiveness. It was a wonderful scene of chaos. It resulted in the two of them missing their school bus. Jim, Peter's dad, had left the house almost an hour earlier for work. Nancy, his mom, was scrambling to get them into the car to drive them to school when she slipped on some ice in their driveway and ended up flat on her back. Can you say pain pills? I couldn't wait!

A neighbor, who just happened to be watching the event from their window, came out to check on her and ended up calling an ambulance. It was a big scene with lots of drama. I love drama. I'm not sure if she broke anything or not, I wasn't concerned about that. What I wanted to know was what would she be bringing home with her from the ER? Hydrocodone ended up being the script du jour. I was hoping for a schedule II like an Oxy or a methadone but I guess she didn't fall hard enough for the really good stuff. But hey, I can work with what we have, and we had Vicodin. She tried them the first night and ended up hugging the toilet so she switched to some OTC stuff which, as long as she didn't get rid of the Vicodin, was fine by me. I had plans for the remaining fifty-eight 7.5 ES's. Big plans!

My relationship with Peter continued to deepen as we used delta-9-tetrahydrocannabinol in increasing amounts to numb the noise of his thoughts and feelings of embarrassment and shame. I love to say the word delta-9-tetrahydrocannabinol. It's almost as long as your alphabet. You usually call the active ingredient in marijuana THC, but its long name is much more fun to say. It's probably better for me if you use THC as it sounds much less scary.

The relationship with Peter did have its moments. We eventually got to a point where we had maxed out the weed. I mean a human can only smoke so much during 24 hours and let's face it, Peter wasn't made of money, even though he was stealing as much as he could from his parents, his grandparents, and his aunts and uncles. You creatures can become very unappreciative of all I do for you. I did for Peter exactly what I promised, took away the feelings. But an interesting thing happens when you don't feel. You become numb. After a while, you don't like that either. Numb is a misnomer. On the surface its means not feeling anything. But not feeling actually feels like something - you call it numb - and it too becomes painful for humans. But don't worry, even when you don't appreciate me I'm still willing to help.

Life sometimes has such a great sense of humor. Right when things with Peter were getting a bit stale, his parents decide to try and connect with a new church. They had left the last one after Peter's bad experience in middle school and several other unpleasant encounters. They dragged Peter and his two younger siblings to a small group family dinner in hopes of developing new friendships at the church. I really wish I could have taken credit for what happened that night, but it was just life working with me. When they got there, the teens were sent to the basement to hang out. Peter recognized the music as he headed down the stairs and figured it was going to be lame, but maybe there would be someone who would want to sneak out and smoke. When Peter stepped off the last step and into the room I could feel the blood drain out of his head – but not in a good way. I'm like what? What did I miss? And there he was, Peter's nightmare in the flesh, the upperclassman who played kissy kissy and much more with Peter that first night of the retreat. Wow – refreshed inspiration that would move Peter to take our relationship to a new level.

He felt like a caged animal. I'm not sure who or what he hated more; the kid who used him for a little sexual recreation, having to spend two hours in the same room with his first kiss, or his parents for putting him in this situation. There was actually another option floating in Peter's mind that I gently kept pushing to the surface. The person he should really be thinking about hating was himself. I mean really. "Why didn't you say no Peter? Why did you let him touch you like that? It's because you liked it! Didn't you! You think you're a big tough guy but you didn't do one thing to try and stop him when he started touching you. You're pathetic." The narrative was working. Peter definitely wasn't numb anymore and he was certainly going to need my help.

The silence in the car during the ride home didn't strike Peter's parents as unusual. What they didn't know was that every cell in Peter's body felt like it was on fire. His mind was racing with so many thoughts, images, and feelings. I thought for a moment that his consciousness might implode like a black hole. If I didn't figure out a way to help him, and soon, I was expecting a seventy-two hour stay in the bed and breakfast floor at the regional hospital. My suggesting that he needed to consider HIS role in the whole retreat sex encounter is one of my classic strategies. If I can foster even a hint of self-blame, and nurture it along, it will blossom into a full bouquet of shame. It truly is a masterpiece not unlike those created by Da Vinci or Raphael. In much the same way as they laid down their pallet of colors in perfect order and timing on their canvas, I select and mix your thoughts and float them from the depths of your memory in just the perfect sequence and timing to produce the shame that is my life's blood. Timing is essential. I doubt any of them consciously realized that next week would be the one year anniversary of the church retreat.

Arriving home around 9:45 that evening, Peter quickly dismissed himself to go upstairs to his bedroom to play an online game. No matter how hard he tried to get into the game I made sure the images and feelings from that night a year ago played in his mind. He was reliving the event. It started with emotional confusion followed by the sensation of being touched. The feeling of panic came next. His body felt paralyzed. He knew he should stop the boy but, for some reason couldn't "or didn't want to," I casually added into his thoughts. He gave up on the game around 1:00 a.m. and headed down to the kitchen to get something to drink, anything to avoid lying down to go to sleep. His mom had been in bed for hours and his dad was fast asleep "watching" a late night talk show in the living room. It wasn't that Peter didn't want to sleep, he just couldn't stand all the thoughts that raced through his head the second he would put it on his pillow, the same pillow he had taken on the retreat, the same pillow he had his head on when the upperclassman reached into his sleeping bag and…Will it ever stop he screamed in his head? "NO!" I answered. He may have meant it to be a rhetorical question but I thought I should answer anyway.

As he opened the cupboard door to get a glass, I directed his attention to the small green bottle that had been sitting in a wicker basket on the counter next to the phone. It had crossed his vision almost every day for the past three weeks ever since his mom had fallen on the ice. "You're in pain," I whispered. "They're pain pills, they come from the pharmacy, they're made in a sterile safe place, they're safe, your mom even used them." Peter opened the bottle and gently tapped it against his hand to free two of the tablets. "There are so many in the bottle no one would ever know. Just try…" before I could finish our thought, he had popped two 750 ES's into his mouth and washed them down. Even though they seemed like large pills, he decided to take two because they were only good for four hours and he didn't want to wake up in the middle of the night, even though it already was the middle of the night. I didn't fault his logic – I actually kind of liked it. Man did we sleep well that night.

The way you creatures look at your world is confusing. Peter wouldn't eat a potato chip if it had fallen on the floor, yet he'll take ground up hemp shavings that have been cut, unbeknownst to him, with clippings from a compost pile mixed with a little oregano, light it on fire, and suck it into his lungs. He won't even put oregano on his pizza, but whatever, in the end it all works for me. It's all about avoiding pain. And there's nothing like an opioid analgesic to help you stop feeling pain, or anything else for that matter.

ANTON & SUSAN

For Anton, life would never be the same. I made sure of it. When you kill a little girl just before the birthday party for your twin girls it kind of puts a damper on things. The ER felt like a morgue. Everyone was transported to the same hospital. The first of many racing thoughts started through his mind – "What have I done?" – Which I resonated repeatedly. Hey, I'm just trying to help. It progresses an important question. Susan's parents were at their home for the twin's party when all this happened so she was able leave and come to the hospital. Right after she asked the question, "Are you OK?" She followed up with, "What happened?" But that isn't what he heard. What he heard was, "What have you done!" I jumped in to help by reminding Anton that he had just killed a little girl, just in case he had forgotten. When they arrived home the whole awkward scene was repeated with Susan's parents. The entire day was priceless. It reminded me of that movie The Wizard of Oz when the tornado hit and Dorothy wakes up in Oz and the images go from black and white to vibrant color. Anton wasn't in Kansas anymore, but in my version of the story, there isn't a yellow brick road and the witch wins. I love those little monkeys, the way they swoop in a carry people away.

The first year after the little girl's death was a tug of war for Anton. Everyone kept telling him it was an accident, but I kept telling him the truth, especially at night when it was quiet. Ssshhhh....Anton's sleeping. He's dreaming and it's time for me to whisper my lines..."How could I not see a RED car in the middle of the road? I SHOULD have seen it! Was I looking at the CD changer? What was I looking at? I SHOULD HAVE SEEN IT! It's my FAULT! I KILLED her!" While I value creativity, in this case I stuck to the script because it was working so well. We could all feel it. The clock was ticking down. I love it when life works with me to stack one anniversary date on top of another. It makes them all so easy for you to remember. You, not me. I never forget. From the moment of impact and the imprinting of the little girl's face into Anton's memory the clock began counting down from 17,520 hours — tick tock tick tock. When it hit zero his twins would be the exact same age as the girl he killed - five. It would be one of those extra special anniversary dates. And from that point on, the clock would begin moving forward marking each new milestone experience of his twins and how he had so carelessly stolen those moments from the little girl and her parents. SHAME on him!

The next few years seem to drag on and the twins birthday's came and went with little visible fanfare. Anton and Susan worked hard to portray an image of normalcy to their family, friends, neighbors, and most importantly — at least for me — themselves. Normal is such an easy construct to use against humans. You have within you this competing desire to be both special and normal, but you don't have a working understanding or concept of either. What is normal? What is special? They're whatever I choose to tell you they are, and you believe me. Normal is something you strive to get back to, but when you were there you were secretly hoping things would change. And then there's special. Whenever you're struggling with what I need you to do, I just tell you your situation is special and that's why you're justified in following my lead. Susan's strategy to achieve a state of normal was to ignore it, with "it" being reality. She did this by not talking about "it" with anyone, which was great because I knew that while she wasn't talking about it (the painful reality they had experienced) she was definitely thinking about it, pretty much constantly. She was so angry, but was using every ounce of her physical and emotional strength to not show it, which was strength she was not using against me. The object of her anger continually changed. She hated Anton for not paying attention when he was driving the day of the twin's birthday. He was always screwing with either the XM radio or his cell phone and she was always yelling at him to watch the road. Everything she was experiencing was his fault. Except for on the days when she was angry at herself for sending him to the store in the first place. If she hadn't forgotten to pick up the napkins and juice at the store two days earlier this nightmare wouldn't be happening. The only other reprieve for Anton from

Susan's anger was when it was directed at God. Ultimately, you humans blame him for everything, which is fine by me. It's a great system, he causes your pain and I relieve your pain, it's a match made in….well you know the place.

Anton was storing his grief as well. I was proud of him. He threw himself into his work and avoided anything pleasurable because he and I both knew that he needed to be punished, at least during this phase of our relationship. The great thing about stored grief is that it ferments into my favorite human feeling. Remember? Shame. My relationship with Anton was ripening. With the twins fourth birthday last month we were now on the home stretch. It would be just 8,040 hours to go until our special anniversary.

~ Speaking of anniversaries, don't you just love a good romance? That's really what humans have with me. You have a romantic relationship with me, the love of your life, the one, and ONLY ONE, who understands you, who listens to you without judgment – unless a little judgement would serve my purpose. I'm the one who saves you from all the bad stuff. Bad stuff does happen, but we all know that the bad stuff isn't my fault. It's just the way life is. Truth be told I'm the one who rescues you from having to feel all the bad stuff. I find it so cute when my humans think they have to protect me. It's flattering when I see your devotion to me, but really, I deserve it. No one else is going to save your sorry butt from all the pain in this world. You couldn't survive without me, but it is still cute when you try to protect me.

13

PETER

Clueless Nancy, that's what Peter and I called his mom. Surprisingly, she finally did get a clue one day. It was a Friday morning and she was cleaning up the kitchen after everyone had left for work and school. Every couple of months she would sort through the basket next to the phone that always seemed to be the dumping ground for note pads, pens, receipts, hand-lotion, vitamins, and the occasional doctor's script. She began pulling everything out of the basket, checking the receipts and throwing them out, then she pulled out the green script bottle she had gotten about two months ago when she fell in the driveway. As she grabbed it she had a flashback to how nauseous she felt when she took them. It was a big bottle, something didn't feel right. The feel, the sound, it was almost empty. Even though it was obvious she opened the bottle to confirm her suspicion. There were just nine pills left in the bottle. Her mind began to race. Who was taking them? She had three options, her husband Jim or one of the two kids. She couldn't believe this was happening and found it hard to even imagine that one of her family members could be taking her prescription. Pain pills, drugs, it seemed surreal in her mind.

She immediately called Jim at work. He was in a meeting and she got his voice mail. "Hey Jim, any idea where all the Vicodin went that were sitting by the phone for the past two months?" She didn't actually say that, she just told him they had a problem and he needed to call her right way. She kept telling herself there had to be a logical explanation for the missing pills. Maybe they somehow spilled on the floor and then someone threw them all out, except for the nine that were still in the bottle. She desperately wanted to come up with a reasonable explanation. Finally Jim called back. "There were pills by the phone?" She couldn't believe he didn't remember that she had been given the script when she had fallen. Needless to say, she didn't suspect Jim. She also couldn't imagine it was Karen, or Peter for that matter. It had to be one of their friends that had been in their house.

After all, if one her kids was using drugs, which sounded ridiculous in her head as she thought it, she would know. She decided her and Jim would discuss it with the kids in the morning to try and determine which of their friends had taken her script.

Individuals like Peter, who are dedicated to me, possess extreme attention to detail when it comes to things important to us. My solution to your pain, or any other problem you're experiencing, is to connect you with the vital resources needed to successfully relieve your pain. These resources are essential to our literal well being. They need to be protected from those that don't appreciate and understand their value. Peter arrived home late Friday afternoon after school. He dropped his stuff in his room and he headed for the kitchen. As he rounded the corner from the dinning room and entered the kitchen, his eyes scanned the basket next to the phone with a passing glance. He immediately noticed the missing green bottle but continued straight to the refrigerator without missing a beat. He grabbed something to drink and headed to the living room, again glancing back to confirm the pill bottle was missing. His heart began to pound in his chest. After setting his drink down in the living room, he headed back to his bedroom. He shut his door and then quietly pulled a box of old Wii game controllers from his closet. He pulled one of the controllers from the box that had a telltale scratch on it that only he recognized. He flipped it over and removed the cover for the battery. He then pulled a small plastic bag from within the controller. Two 750 mg Vicodin could be seen in the bag. He just needed to know for sure that they were still there. He quickly returned them to the safety of their hiding place and placed the box back in the corner of his closet.

As he returned to the living room, he began to run through his contingency plan. The bottle had been there this morning before he left for school. He started telling himself that his mom had probably just moved it into the shoe box she kept in their bedroom closet with all the other old scripts. Both of his parents were now home so he couldn't check. Neither of them said anything to him about the bottle and both seemed to be acting relatively normal.

He had removed four of the pills the day before leaving nine in the bottle. He had stashed the two in the Wii controller the week before.

He'd been debating taking the bottle, thinking no one would notice, and now regretted that he hadn't. This could potentially work out even better he began to think. She never checks the shoe box and he could just remove the whole bottle or better yet replace the remaining pills with a similar looking generic, or over the counter. Peter had started to panic about a week earlier as the pills began to dwindle. I tried to reassure him that I would take care of him and provide a plan. On the other hand, sometimes panic is a great motivator and you just need to let it build and then leverage the energy. I always want to keep my options open.

Peter got up at his usual time for a Saturday. He figured at some point, his mom would run some errands and he could safely search for the missing bottle. As he entered the kitchen, his sister and parents were in the dinning room eating breakfast. It only took a microsecond glance - the Vicodin bottle was on the dinning room table next to one of the cereal boxes. "Peter, we need you to come in here. There's something we need to talk about." It was his mom. His heart rose up into his throat. He mentally began to prepare for the interrogation.

To his shock, surprise, and general relief, his mom and dad started talking about he and his sister's friends and if they thought any of them might have a drug problem. When Karen asked why, her mom picked up the script bottle and explained how a considerable amount of the pills had disappeared and they were suspecting one of their friends. Peter couldn't take his eyes off the bottle. He could hear the pills shifting in the bottle. His mom was still talking but he didn't hear anything she was saying. "Peter, what about Andy? Sometimes he seems a little out of it. Do you think he may have taken them?" When he heard his name he snapped back to reality. At first he said no, but as the discussion continued he realized that if they eliminated all of their friends as suspects, that left only him and Karen. Upon this realization, he changed his position and selected a classmate that neither of his parents were all that familiar with and put him out there as the potential thief. The debate then shifted to whether the suspects parents should be contacted.

The discussion, which seemed to Peter to have lasted hours, started to wind down after about twenty minutes. The whole time, Peter never let the bottle out of his sight. Even when he was making eye contact with his parents, he was tracking the green bottle with his peripheral vision. His primary concern was not losing track of the bottle. But how he would connect with the remaining nine pills at this point was going to be problematic, but he at least needed to know where they were.

The next words out of his mom's mouth seemed as if they were on a time delay. It totally caught Peter off guard and she was moving across the room before the words registered in his brain. "Even if we never find out for sure whether that kid took them, I'm going to make sure it doesn't happen again! I should have done this a month ago." Peter began to panic. "Where is she going?" I asked. Peter knew she was headed for the bathroom. "The bathroom? Peter you got to stop her!" "Mom what are you doing?" You could hear the panic in his voice. "Mom what are you doing?" Her response lit his brain on fire, "I'm going to flush them!" she said. "Mom you can't! Wait! You're not suppose to do that! Wait!" He said even louder.

Peter was in total survival mode at this point and had caught up to her in the hallway and was struggling to get in front of her to block her path. His dad and sister sat stunned at the table as the drama moved down the hall. His mom was fumbling with the child proof cap as she entered the bathroom with Peter in hot pursuit pulling on her arm. "PETER! What's wrong? Stop it!" Her yelling momentary stunned him and he froze. She had the cap off by now and lifted the lid to the toilet. The pills slid out of the bottle from a height of not more than twenty inches. Within a second they hit the water. "NO!" He and I screamed. As her hand touched the handle on the toilet tank I screamed into Peter's brain, "GRAB IT GRAB IT GRAB IT GRAAAAAB IT!!!!!!!!!" Without even so much as a second thought he plunged his hand down into the water to rescue the Vicodin at the bottom of the toilet bowl. His hand hit the water the same time his mom flushed the toilet. It was a photo finish, it would only be a moment before we knew who won.

His dad and sister finally joined us in the bathroom for family time to hear Nancy repeatedly yelling her son's name as if she was trying to summon him back to their reality. What they didn't understand *was that Peter was now firmly in my reality, not theirs. His fist tightly securing four of the damp pills, his eyes were fixed on the toilet bowl as the tank refilled, he was like a stone statue, he didn't appear to be breathing. A series of phrases could be simultaneously heard echoing in his brain as if being broadcast from another galaxy, "What's going on? What's wrong? Peter look at me!"*

Peter was at the edge. Deep inside his brain he was having a conversation with himself. I was there listening. He was moving through the list of items humans deem essential to survival; food, water, oxygen. He kept going over the list in his subconscious. He was partially pulled back to your reality when he felt someone touch the fist that held his oxygen. He was scared, unsure of what was going to happen next. "Breath." I gently whispered in the deepest part of his brain. With the speed of a lightening bolt Peter popped the four damp pills into his mouth and swallowed them. It was now clear to everyone in the room who had won. The moment was priceless, a bit soggy and bitter tasting, but still priceless.

14
JULIE

Julie pretty much devoted herself to volleyball and track during her high school years, which to her parent's great pleasure resulted in a nominal athletic scholarship to a small, but respectable, university in Colorado. For the past 4 years, since the infamous morning when her brother walked in on her and her uncle, she had abstained from anything and everything sexual and had thrown herself into sports and academics. Those daily early morning runs were killers. It wasn't so much that she was trying to improve her time as she was just running to get away from what was chasing her in her mind. Run run run...I personally thought it was a bit ridiculous. It's kind of like the opposite of a cat chasing its tail. I went along for the ride because I knew she would eventually get tired of running. I also knew when she did, she would turn to me to save her from the pain that she had been so desperately trying to stay one step ahead of.

Julie's parents, while slightly apprehensive at the thought of leaving their little girl as she was standing outside of her dorm waving goodbye to them, felt confident in their daughter's ability to continue along the same successful path she had followed in high school. The fact that it was now legal to use cannabis in Colorado wasn't a big concern for them. Julie looked down on those who used it and prided herself on not associating with "those" people. I was fine with that as I had plenty of tools at my disposal. The first invitation to a party came that evening before her parents were even an hour out of town on their way back home. It was Thursday, and classes were scheduled to begin the following Monday. While that first kegger wasn't anything for the record books – I think Julie drank one beer – I rejoiced at the change I was beginning to see in her. We didn't run Friday morning.

I don't think she could put her finger on it but something had changed inside her. She no longer had the emotional energy to run from her pain and it was beginning to overtake her. She went to her classes and athletic practices, but she wasn't the brightest or fastest anymore. She couldn't fully contain her feelings or her thoughts the way she could back home. College was different. The structure provided by the presence of her parents was no longer there. The classes were bigger, longer, and more intense. Guys were hitting on her and the overall environment was much more sexually charged, especially in the dorms. All of it was generating confusing flashbacks of her uncle. She had mixed emotions over the attention from the guys. It was both exciting and aggravating. Then I started the dreams. They weren't nightmares, I didn't need to scare, I just wanted to add a bit more confusion into her thoughts. She didn't like thinking about what her uncle had done to her. When she did, I would gently reminder her that she was a more than willing partner. Uncle John was only going along with what she really wanted. I always try to help people keep my facts straight.

She was majoring in business and quickly settled into a routine. The school was on a semester system and Julie was taking seventeen credits. She was taking two prerequisite business classes, a freshman English class, a basic history class, and a PE class. Her classes were spread evenly throughout the week with the exception of Thursday, which was her busiest day due to volleyball practice and a special English lab that was required of all freshman. The classes were harder then she expected. High school academics had come easy for her and she never had to put in much effort. College was different, she was having to put in a lot more work just to keep up. She was shocked when her first official grade on a paper for one of her business courses was a C. It was her first ever.

She had met a handful of her fellow classmates and would frequently join them for lunch or dinner in the dining hall. The conversation never got very deep. It was a couple weeks after midterm exams that our relationship really began to blossom. Low grades, fear of possible academic probation, and the thought that her scholarship could be in jeopardy sent Julie running in my direction. Her increasing sense of failure was becoming overwhelming. She had disappointed her uncle, her brother, and her parents. The only reason her parents didn't know the truth about what a disappointment she had been was because she had been using every ounce of her strength to maintain the façade of being the perfect daughter. Secrets and image control are two of my favorite things. They drain the physical and emotional energy from humans like nothing else. Combine that with the soul sucking isolation they create and it's my perfect storm. After the Saturday morning volleyball clinic fiasco four years earlier, she had adopted the rule that silence was her safest strategy – OK, I probably helped with that. Anytime she would even begin to entertain the idea of sharing our secret about Uncle John, or the intense loneliness she was feeling, I would jump into her thoughts and walk her through the soul crushing condemnation she would have to endure from everyone she might turn to for solace. I made sure she understood that she had nowhere to turn - but to me.

It was Friday, which meant it was favorite pink sweater day. If anything, Julie was predictable. She had finished her one morning class and was back in her dorm room. Her room was on the fifth floor with an East facing window. In high school she would always run before school so she like the early morning sun coming through the window, but not so much these days. Her dorm had just been built just a few years earlier so the rooms, while small, where relatively nice. Her roommate, also a freshman, had an ROTC scholarship that kept her busy so they rarely saw each other. The dining hall would stop serving in twenty minutes. Julie didn't have much of an appetite, she felt empty, but not hungry. She decided to skip lunch. She also decided to blow off her afternoon classes, what was the point, she was a failure. Well technically her academic efforts were resulting in low grades, but I encouraged her to step up and own her failure. It was who she was – it was her identity. Some call it shame, I call it the truth. Her world was collapsing like a black hole and I was cultivating her sense of claustrophobia - her sense of panic was growing slowly. I was feeling a bit bored and thinking maybe we should not waste the beautiful fall afternoon and go for a walk. It was like she had read my mind, which was a bit strange for me, as she headed out of her room toward the elevator.

The university had been founded in the early 1900's and had four original, red brick buildings at the center of the campus. They had been restored and were now used for administrative offices. The campus had expanded over the years with newer buildings reflecting the decade in which they were built. To the West the campus butted up against an old residential neighborhood, most of which had been built prior to the 1960's. The neighborhood had been losing the battle to the gradual expansion of the school over the years. The majority of the campus dorms were on the West side of campus as well. As the school would acquire the old homes, they would renovate the usable ones to rent out to fraternities or sororities. Julie's feeling of claustrophobia was increasing her sense of urgency to get out of the building. She regretted taking the elevator and not running the stairs. She headed for the closest exit as she stepped out of the elevator. It faced West. The mix of the cool fresh air with the warmth of the sun provided a brief moment of relief, but nothing like I could provide her.

She wasn't more than five minutes into her walk when she recognized the two gentlemen on the porch of the renovated victorian style home. She had been there once before at the beginning of the semester. They smiled and said hi, which was the first inkling of human affection she had felt all day. She made an impulse decision to join them on the porch and shortly after accepted their offer to go inside where it was warmer. It was a beautifully foyer. She loved the design and texture of the ceiling. The way the sunlight entered the room just felt relaxing. A crystal hanging in the window created a subtle pattern of colors. She would lay and watch the colors float across the ceiling as she waited for her alarm to go off again after hitting the snooze button. As she gained more consciousness the panicked thought, "What time is it?" jumped into her head. She relaxed when she realized it was Saturday. "What happened to Friday? Why is my pajama shirt pulling against my neck? It became even more uncomfortable now that she noticed. As she began to pull herself from under the covers the panic returned and rushed over her like an ice cold ocean wave. She was still wearing her pink sweater, but she had it on backwards! She attempted to clear her mind and focus, but there was nothing there. Her panic increased.

The past eighteen-twenty hours was mixed up bits and blurry pieces at best. Even I don't completely remember all of it. She fought to remember but her head was pounding. She vaguely remembered stepping onto the porch of a house. She couldn't decide in her mind if it was a dream or a memory. Then there were images of being inside the house, but really nothing after that. She could see faces but they weren't clear and she couldn't put names to any of them. I remembered the vodka. The C_2H_6O (alcohol) from her first three drinks entered her blood stream with her stomach being empty and quickly flowed to her brain. There it interacted with the gamma–aminobutyric acid receptors in the hippocampus area of her brain to not only produce a wonderful sedation, but also a complete memory blackout - oops. It was now 9:48 am on Saturday morning and her last clear memory was from some nineteen hours earlier. Her heart began to race uncontrollably as she realized she wasn't wearing her bra. I told her it was no big deal and besides, she needed to be focused on what was important. Me.

15
ANTON & SUSAN

It was like the sound of thunder on a clear day, totally out of place. It actually caught me off guard. Anton had just walked back into his office at Image Tech after a meeting for a software development project. He wasn't breathing! He fell into his desk chair. He was clutching his chest as if trying to make it work. I'm not sure if it was me or Anton that was yelling in his head, "BREATHE!" He managed to pull his tie lose – it didn't help. His heart was racing and he was beginning to sweat. In the midst of the panic, he could feel the sweat slowly running down his back - it sent chills through his body. He was finally able to suck in a breath. It hurt like nothing he had felt before – but now he couldn't exhale and he felt like he was drowning in his own air - he willed himself to push it out and take another. His mind raced, "Am I dying, is this a heart attack, should I call 911?" The room lost all of its color, everything was grey. After the third breath made it into his lungs the shaking started. "WHAT'S HAPPENING?" He screamed in his head! He wasn't actually saying any words, I was trying not to laugh because he was making this funny wheezing sound as he tried to breath. His office door had shut behind him so he was in the room alone. He stumbled to pull his cell phone from his suit pocket but was shaking so bad he dropped it. He thought about trying to make it to the door, but his legs were numb. That's because all of the blood had left his limbs as his body prepped itself to avoid going into shock.

After about five minutes – which seemed like hours to Anton - the shaking began to subside and his breathing began to slow down. Anton still didn't know what had just happened, but I did. OK, so it took me a minute just because it caught me off guard, Anton had just experienced his first official panic attack. I know you think I'm inappropriate, but I just couldn't stop smiling! We get to go see the doctor! And Clonazepam is at the top of my wish list. It's my most favorite benzodiazepine. Its more common name is Klonopin. It's got all the sedation of alcohol without having to get up to constantly pee. And it's so much more convenient than alcohol - you can carry a whole bottle of seventy - one hundred in your pocket like nobody's business. Ever try and carry a case of beer in your pocket?

Anton didn't tell Susan about his near death panic attack he had in his office. He didn't tell her about the three others that had happened in the months that followed either. Anton and Susan hadn't talked about anything meaningful since he had killed the little girl. She knew he had seen his doctor but he had passed it off as a physical required by his work. He told her the new medication was something the doctor recommended for work related stress. And just as I had predicted, the doctor gave him my favorite - Klonopin. And just in time – not to save Anton – I could care less about his stupid panic attacks - I'm talking about my plan to deepen my relationship with him and his family. I didn't just want him – I wanted Susan too and I was putting everything in place to introduce Susan to the power of "vitamin K" as well as a few of my other tools. But I'll get to that a little bit later.

Remember that special anniversary I had been waiting for? The twins fifth birthday was now just three weeks away. This would be an epic event, but one that would be missed by everyone in the family. Or at least no one would speak of it or fully recognize its significance. I'm not talking about the twins fifth birthday, but the fact that Daniel & Chanel were now the same age as dead Sarah, the cute little blond in the back of the red car.

Orchestration is a complex art form no matter what the medium. It requires finesse, timing, and all the right ingredients. Greatness is demonstrated by those able to create something powerfully beautiful with the simplest of ingredients. I take relationships, circumstances, unique life events, accidents, traumas, rejection, loneliness, and disappointment and use each of them in combination to secure my place of prominence in your life. It is pretty impressive. But so often you miss the powerful subtleties of how I weave each of these things together for maximum human impact. The fact that Anton killed the little girl on his twins' birthday was priceless. That the "accident" took place on one of the main roads in their neighborhood was frosting on my cake. Cake – that reminds me, I need to get back and fill you in on porky Karen in a minute. Anton had developed an awkward alternative driving route to avoid the intersection of our conception, as I like to call it. I don't give him a rough time about it though; the extra minute or two added to the drive just gives us more time to think about why we're going the long way. That extra time to think helped Anton to max out his dose of Klonopin within just four weeks of when we started the script.

It was at this same time that Susan came around and recognized her need for me. Maintaining the façade of normal had finally taken its full toll on her and she had become an emotional black hole – stuffing and sucking in every negative painful feeling. Telling herself over and over, "Doesn't matter." She had been working as hard as she could to convince her parents and her siblings that her relationship with Anton was fine and that every time she looked at her twins she didn't think about dead Sarah and what her parents must be feeling right at that moment. I loved that thought because I could play spin-the-bottle as to who we would blame. Some days it was Anton for not paying attention, other days it was her for sending him to the store, and now more recently we added dead Sarah's parents for running that red light, "Those idiots, they've ruined my life!" And then there was always God. On my best days they all got blamed. That, of course, was my ultimate goal because when you blame everyone, you stand alone; well except for me...I'm your only friend who is ready and willing to bring you comfort and relief from your pain. And Susan's emotional pain was about to crush her.

I've been thinking about getting a cape, I'm just not sure what color. The super hero motif appeals to me, except for the tights, they just don't look comfortable. Needless to say, I swooped in at the last possible moment to rescue Susan from the emotional black hole that was sucking the life out of her. It had been a long day and the twins had been crabby most of the evening and had finally gone to sleep after a prolonged battle. Anton was in his man cave being comforted by me. By the way if you had missed this point – I'm omnipresent. Susan and I were in the kitchen. She was standing at the sink staring out the window contemplating how numb could feel so painful. I was staring at Anton's bottle of Klonopin that he had so carelessly, yet *conveniently, left on the counter. Finally she looked down. "It can't make things any worse," I said in my best Susan voice inside her head. She picked up the bottle as if to read the label, "If anyone's under stress in this family, it's me!" Her thought threw me for a minute because she said it before I did! Susan had taken the ball and was off and running, now all I had to do was steer, but we both knew where she was going. I suggested we pour a glass of wine, she agreed. I suggested we use the wine to wash down one of Anton's pills, she agreed. We then celebrated another one of my birthdays! It was a small party, just one Klonopin and a glass of wine, but that painful numbness she had been feeling was also gone. OK, technically it wasn't actually gone as in not in existence anymore – but she couldn't "feel" it anymore and if you read the fine print that's exactly what I do, sort of, I make the pain go away, for a while.*

16

JOHN

John had always been careful when it came to driving. His blood alcohol content on his first DUI was just at the edge of the legal limit. His low blood alcohol level, combined with his lack of any other legal issues and a good lawyer, resulted in minimal inconvenience for me. The second, which happened several years later, occurred while he was on a business trip out of state. The nature of the trip forced him to risk endangering our relationship by driving because he felt he had to get back to meet a family "obligation." Bureaucracy and poor state legal coordination helped me out, and the legal system never connected the dots to the first DUI. He blamed being a day late getting home on a freak snow storm – his family and friends didn't even think twice about it. His third, however, didn't go as well. He had passed out while stopped at a red light. His blood alcohol content more than twice the legal limit. The real issue was a new national data base that allowed local law enforcement to discover DUI number 2, there was no way John could avoid the annoyance of "treatment." I wasn't worried though. Barring what humans refer to as a miracle, my relationship with John was sealed to the end.

I hate tough choices, John did too. Ninety days in jail, without what we needed, or several weeks of intensive outpatient torture. I opted for the torturous treatment. I knew I could handle it. We'd just have to endure some idiot therapist poking around John's childhood asking him, "So John, why do you hate your parents?" Not only could I handle it, I wanted it, bring it on! Poke away! John had been keeping that secret for over thirty-five years. John's dad couldn't stop his mom from drinking and he hated him for it. There were days as a small child when he would cry for hours in panic because his mom would be passed out and he couldn't wake her – he hated her for that. His loser older brother checked out of the family and left him alone and defenseless. The only two people he remembers getting any attention from were sexual predators, which he himself had become. And all of these thoughts I just shared with you...were never shared with another human being...just me.

Treatment lasted for two months, I can hold my breath longer than that. "Where do they find these people? You're nothing like them!" I started playing that phrase on a constant loop in John's head. John didn't realize it but he was actually just like them. They were my people. Each one of them. Even though they were united in their pain, I made sure each of them continued to feel and stay isolated, misunderstood, and persecuted. Sitting through treatment was harder for John than it was for me, I pretty much slept through it. When we weren't at treatment or work we were at home watching porn. DUI number three resulted in twenty-four months of probation. John had to regularly check in with a probation officer and he was subject to no notice visits at his apartment where he could be required to take a breathalyzer. The rhythm of the unannounced evening PO visits became predicable and we would sneak a few drinks after the visits, but that was our little secret. As a result of the legal issues, John lost his license. But fortunately he held onto his job and lived close enough to both his work and a grocery store that I was able to survive.

John's mom was very supportive. She was still completely devoted to me and understood us. She wanted to protect her son just like I did. Well maybe not in the exact same way, but she didn't want anything bad to happen to him. His dad had long given up fighting me and was now an ally. He was now serving me with the respect I deserve. Although it wasn't always pretty, the three of them generally worked well together in making sure I had what I needed. In return, I provided John and his mother the relief they so desperately desired. John's dad didn't want my help. And that was fine as I needed him to stay focused helping the other two. Life was good for me.

17

KAREN & PETER

Virtually all of my stories intersect. Everyone knows at least a few of my people, you just don't know that you know them. For the hundreds of painful thoughts and feelings that race through people's heads, it's rare that even one of them gets shared with anyone else. When families do finally become aware of my presence it usually has an apocalyptic feel to it. Ever see one of those video clips where they show the moon slowly moving in front of the sun to create a total eclipse event? Everything goes dark in the middle of the day and you think the world is ending. That's kind of what happened after the bobbing for Vicodin episode with Porky Karen's brother Peter. The world appeared to be ending for her parents and the "Peter crisis" totally eclipsed Karen's existence.

My theory was the only way we were going to be noticed was to make ourselves bigger. It had been just over six months since her last visit to the doctor. The red LED numbers on the scale zipped up to 250 instantaneously. Karen was beginning to wonder how high the numbers went. Her doctor had recommended a cocktail of bupropion and naltrexone. The first is an antidepressant and the second was supposed to decrease her appetite. The doc also wanted her to attend a nutrition class. That just made us hungry. To be honest, each pound felt like a hundred pounds to her. "Why can't I stop?" was the thought that continually played in her head. She hated her weight and how her body looked, but loved eating. She felt pulled to food, driven to eat like she was driven to breath, she simply could not overrule her desire to eat. The doctor, the school nurse and school counselor had talked with her about her risk for developing type II diabetes. The school nurse had given her pamphlets about it and wanted her and her parents to come in for nutrition counseling. "Not now!" or "I'll look at it later!" were the most common responses from her parents any time she tried to bring it up. "Can't you see we have to take care of this thing with your brother?" "This thing" would ring in her head. She wanted to scream

"What about my THING!" But figured it would only be met with, "Not now!" She was alone, except for me.

Human families are so easy to dismember. It's all about the "ates." Separate, isolate, denigrate, and humiliate. Shake, stir, wait five-minutes and you all go your separate ways. I don't have to divide in order to conquer – you guys take care of that for me – you're all so helpful!

I pretty much had porky Karen set on auto pilot for the next decade. As I already said, food isn't the most glamorous of my mediums, but it's easy and takes very little effort on my part. Between all your carb and sugar loaded foods, combined with all the advertising, it really is a piece of cake. Karen was on track to eat herself into oblivion. I'll come back to her later. My work with her brother Peter, the toilet diver, was much more interesting at this point.

It's so entertaining to watch family members try to explain their relative's behavior to others when their loved one is in love with me. The phone call was awkward to say the least.

Pastor: "Now what exactly is he taking the medicine for? Did he get hurt?"

Nancy: "He didn't get hurt, I did, but I wasn't taking the pain meds, Peter has been taking them."

Pastor: "Why would he be doing that? Jim said something happened with the toilet. Did Peter fall? Is that why he was taking the pain medication?"

Nancy: "No he didn't fall! He took the Vicodin out of the toilet when I was trying to get rid of it!"

Pastor: "He what? That isn't what Jim said. Is Jim there at the house? To be honest we've never had this kind of issue with any of the other kids in the youth group. Has Peter been bringing these drugs to the youth group? I'm not sure what to...I'll try and get ahold of the youth pastor and have him stop over and talk to Peter."

Nancy: "Peter said he doesn't want to see him."

Pastor: "Why wouldn't he want to talk to the youth pastor?

Nancy: "I DON'T KNOW!"

At this point clueless Nancy was using the same nickname for her pastor that I use for her. She also wished she never made the phone call. Peter ended up being mandated by his parents to do six weeks of "counseling" with Pastor Jake. He was the youth pastor at the their church. At the suggestion of some of their friends, his parents also made him go and speak with a drug counselor. They said it was part of his punishment.

Pastor Jake was two years into his first position as a youth pastor and his initial excitement for youth ministry was starting to wane. He was updating his resume when the senior pastor called to tell him to connect with Peter and straighten him out. Jake pulled his notes from his pastoral care class he had taken at bible college. He had a whole 3 pages on, "Youth, Alcohol and Addiction." It was three pages because he wrote big and always skipped lined in his notes. As I've already said, I'm a mystery to virtually all of you and what you think you know about me isn't actually correct.

Just as a side note, while I thrive in the ignorance of humans, I sometimes feel just a little insulted by how shallow you think I am. It's always alcohol with you. You have so little appreciation for the depth and breadth of my palette. Take the benzodiazepine class of drugs for example. I have over thirty shades of medications to work with just in that one class of drugs, but all you ever think about is alcohol. You can't even begin to comprehend, or appreciate, what I'm doing with video gaming or social media. I have one hundred and one plus ways to light up your brain's nucleus accumbens like a Christmas tree, but all you think about is alcohol.

I almost hate to admit it but churches are frequently one of my best allies and sources of support - not that I need any help. They pride themselves on how they help "Those people." They offer a space in their basement for "Those people." Sometimes they even hire someone to work with "Those people." For much of their lives my people keep me a secret because they believe no one will understand our special relationship, which is true. Once the news of our special relationship is revealed to the world, or the church, the sorting and isolation begins. My people, are immediately labeled "Those people." But as I've already shared with you, I thrive upon isolation, so thanks for the help!

It was a toss up over which one of them, Peter or Pastor Jake, felt more tortured throughout the six weeks. Each week was a dance of tangents. Pastor Jake wasn't really sure where to start and Peter fended off the majority of his attempts to engage with vague commentary or the posing of unanswerable theological questions. I think it was in week six that Peter briefly contemplated asking Jake the famous question of "why." It was actually a string of "why" and "what" questions. Why did God allow that pervert upperclassman to do that to me? Why didn't Pastor Jake protect him? What had Peter done in his young life that made God hate him so much? And about eight - ten more variations on the same theme. But the minute he started to think about asking that first question I reminded him of two important facts; he could trust no one except me and what happened to him that night was his own fault. He had no one to blame but himself. But if he wanted to blame God, Pastor Jake, his parents, the upperclassman, or whoever else he could come up with, I was fine with that too. But he just couldn't talk about it with anyone. Those were my rules.

Meeting with the drug counselor was only for a single session and was no problem at all. When it comes to me, that is Addiction, I'm the expert and I know how to navigate each and every threat to my existence. Substance abuse treatment has very strict confidentiality laws designed to protect my privacy. Well technically it's your privacy but as I've already said this isn't about you, it's about me. The age of consent for substance abuse treatment is thirteen, which meant as long as Peter wasn't planning to hurt himself or someone else the counselor couldn't say a word about what we talked about without Peter signing a release.

18

SUSAN

Susan's first experience with Klonopin was so refreshing. It was like she had been wandering for days in the desert and then discovered an oasis filled with cool water and tons of fresh fruit. We had begun a regular evening relationship that had been continuing for the past fifteen Klonopin, I mean days. I knew we would eventually face a supply crisis with only one Klonopin bottle and two eager humans. I debated whether I should prompt Susan to become more protective of our relationship and start planning ahead, or if I should just let the impending crisis naturally unfold and then surf the chaos. Ever see the news footage of the guy out surfing in the storm waves while everyone else is evacuating because a hurricane is about to do a billion dollars' worth of damage? That's me out surfing! I love storms, but I also love my Klonopin.

Susan was a responsible addict in the making. She was already working on strategies to meet my needs. If Anton could get these things, how hard can it be she thought? She didn't know about Anton's panic attacks, however, and was extremely annoyed when her doctor suggested she take a yoga class to reduce her stress. I have to admit I wasn't all that amused either, but Susan was resourceful and I knew she would come through. We just needed to think. She was also going to need to replace at least a portion of what she had already removed from Anton's bottle.

My followers are always looking for opportunities, and for Susan the opportunity came just the next day. She had plans to go shopping with her friend Maggie that morning and had come into her house because as usual, Maggie was running late. She hated public restrooms so she decided to take advantage of the delay and use Maggie's bathroom. When she got done doing her business, there it was right in front of her, the medicine cabinet, or as I call it, opportunity. How many friends did she have? Each one had a medicine cabinet! Would we get lucky with door number one? As she

61

stared at herself in the mirrored door, she slowly tried to open it. The magnet eventually gave way and the door began to swing open. Her peripheral vision caught the image of her face as she opened the door. It felt like an out of body experience for her as she seemed to be peering behind her own face. She gently searched through the bottles desperately trying to not make noise, while at the same time trying to remember how to put everything back exactly where it was. Susan's heart was pounding - Amitriptyline, _Hydrocortisone_, Amoxicillin, Ibuprofen, Lovastatin, but nothing in the benzo class. Susan had done her research before she went to see her doctor because she knew I wanted benzodiazepines. She wasn't sure about the Amitriptyline, so she Googled it on her smartphone – "Why on earth would Maggie be taking an anti-depressant?" she whispered out loud. She was out of time and needed to get out of the bathroom – but at least now she had a plan of action. It was time to renew old friendships and use each of their bathrooms!

It was like going on the local Parade-of-Homes Tour, only different. Susan was learning more about her friends than she could ever imagine. Much to her surprise and our pleasure – I wasn't actually surprised but it did make me happy –we discovered a treasure trove. It was like being give the keys to a pharmacy. And thanks to Google and her smart phone, Susan learned the new language of the pharmaceutical world and began navigating the green bottles - Fluoxetine, Clonazepam, _Alprazolam_, _Diazepam_, _Lorazepam_ – Susan quickly learned to look for "pam" or "lam" at the end of the name. She also began to note how fast her friends were moving through their scripts and their probable refill dates. It's much less noticeable when you remove 8 or 9 pills from a full 90 count script. My future depended upon her not screwing this up, so I really appreciated her attention to detail.

Susan's pharmaceutical quest was a character building exercise that I had planned for our own good. I had multiple purposes for this phase of her journey. I needed to hone key elements of her life. Stress, anger and shame are a perfect trifecta for keeping me healthy. Each one has multiple flavors and intensities that mix in various amounts to create the equivalent of a culinary masterpiece. Each one interacts with the others, fosters the others, and enhances the experience of the others. I could feel the nervous excitement beginning to build and move through her body as Susan turned down the street where her friend Amanda lived. She was starting to perspire as she pulled into Amanda's driveway. Ahhhh....can't you just feel the norepinephrine beginning to flow across the neurons. Based upon our medicine cabinet recon mission of Amanda's bathroom last week, there was a high probability that we would find a freshly refilled Clonazepam script. The norepinephrine was the precursor to the full up adrenaline rush we were about to experience.

Amanda's house was in a new development and only about half the lots had homes on them. Her husband had just recently started his practice as an optometrist and they had purchased a new home south of Kansas City. She had met Amanda through their church. "How could they afford this place?" she thought as she pulled into the driveway. "Life is so unfair! Even with the wealth of Anton's family, they were facing some significant legal fees as a result of his killing little Sarah. They weren't actually in financial trouble, but I frequently reminded her of where they could have been in life if it hadn't been for the accident. "Focus Susan," I whispered.

After Amanda met her at the door, they began walking towards the back of the home. From the foyer to the kitchen to the media room, everything that was visible was perfect. Even the apparent haphazard placement of accents on end tables was completely scripted. They ended up sitting in the sunroom just off the kitchen. Amanda was talking and Susan was responding with apparent appropriateness, but Susan really had no idea what she was saying or what they were talking about. "Stop staring, calm down, breathe," I was working hard to keep her calm.....Susan's mind was racing a thousand miles per hour – we needed that adrenaline rush to kick in and help her focus. Chitchat, chitchat, blah-blah-blah...so close, but yet so far. Amanda finally broke her unending dialogue to step into the kitchen to get some mundane snack or something – this would be our opportunity. "I'm going to run to the bathroom while you do that," Susan said in her best casual voice. The script was just down the hall in the master bathroom. The challenge would be for Susan to pass the closer guest bathroom to make it to the master bath without being noticed.

As my followers become more devoted to me, one skill that I find so inspiring is their self-serving confidence with which they tackle the tasks required for my care and pleasure. They act with sound belief and devotion. Susan passed by the guest bathroom on the way to the master bedroom without hesitation and quickly enough that it went unnoticed by Amanda who was busy in the kitchen. As she moved through the bedroom and into the bathroom she began to feel her heart pound in her chest as a result of the adrenaline that was now flowing. You're probably thinking she was nervous or scared. She was excited! This was the thrill of the hunt – the anticipation. Was it going to be there? The little green bottle was on the second shelf almost in the exact same spot as last time, which gave Susan pause and made her momentarily nervous. "Didn't she fill it!" raced through her mind. Anticipation was now mixed with fear, and she could feel her pulse in her fingers as she reached for the bottle. She immediately recognized by the weight of the bottle that it was full. It was an almost orgasmic experience as she began to pull the tablets from the bottle and transfer them into a container in her small handbag. Ten tabs were all she was going to take, we couldn't risk getting caught. Apparently Susan's adrenal glands were running a bit low as her hands were now starting to shake. She lost control of the last tab and it dropped into the sink and it began to roll toward the drain – she became so flustered she almost spilled the entire bottle. Fortunately gravity kept them in the bottle and she was able to pull up the drain handle and pinched the pill right at the edge of the drain before it fell.

I was starting to get a little annoyed but also recognized the opportunity before me. "Are you trying to get caught?" I screamed in her head! "Do you think maybe you can make a little more noise….you are such an idiot….can't you do anything right? Every time I give you something to do you screw it up!" You probably don't know this about me but I do great impressions. In this case, I was doing a perfect impression of Susan's mom, right down to her quirky accent – in fact I was doing an exact quote from a time when Susan was eleven and she dropped a set of metal mixing bowls on their kitchen floor and her mom verbally ripped her to shreds. I find that periodic doses of shaming messages are helpful for my people. Most of the time you get them directly from yourself, but sometimes I need to replay those messages in order to maintain the right balance of stress, anger, and shame.

Now it was time for our egress back to the sunroom and Amanda. Susan flushed the toilet and turned on the water for a moment. She pulled herself together and started heading back down the hall all the time rehearsing what her first comments would be to Amanda, who was already back in the sunroom. "I just love the tile combination in your master bath. We're planning to redo our guest bath and want to try and find a similar pattern." That seemed plausible. Susan was developing another one of my essential survival skills – lying. But it's not really a lie if you believe it.

The mundane chitchat continued for about an hour. As we backed out of Amanda's driveway, it was time to tweak the mix. We'd had two helpings of stress, and a small dose of shame, now we needed to add a little anger. I pondered how we should arrive there, and I decided to use a touch of guilt to kick things off. "Stealing from your church friend…could you stoop any lower?" That was all it took to produce a nauseating and overwhelming sense of guilt to wash over "Little Suzie." "Little Suzie, what have you done?" Susan, a.k.a. Little Suzie, felt like she was 5 years old again and could hear her mom's voice ringing in her head, "What have you done?" Suzie would yell back a profanity laced diatribe targeted at her mother, but never out loud, only in her mind. "How dare her….How could he have been so stupid…This is all Anthony's fault!" In an instant, her guilt exploded into anger. This time it was focused on her husband. It really didn't matter to me who the target was; this was my cue to jump into the dialogue. "You're only doing what you have to do to survive – You're the only one holding this family together – give me a break – with everything you have to put up with…who wouldn't need something to help with all the stress." We were now both looking forward to a date with a Klonopin and a tall glass of wine for the evening.

19

JULIE

Julie's dad kept calling and calling. It was getting ridiculous. The guy was so obnoxious - always wanting to tell Julie what to do and when to do it, and then always pointing out when Julie did it wrong. I liked him! Dan, Julie's dad, was what some humans call an ACOA, or Adult Child Of an Alcoholic. I prefer the title Loyal Enablers Meeting My Iconoclastic Needs Gallantly. I call them lemmings for short. Dan and his brother John grew up in a home devoted to me. Sure we had our moments, but I used those moments like the paint on an artist's pallet, playing each moment off the other to achieve my will, just like I was doing at that moment with Julie and her dad. Julie was not only getting annoyed, she was getting scared. It had been two weeks since her blackout. She was pretty sure she recognized a guy from the frat house in one of her large lecture classes, but was afraid to make eye contact with him, or with anyone for that matter. Her paranoia would soon be off the charts, which is why she needed me. I could help her with that.

Dad's paranoia was also going up. Julie didn't make her usual call the previous weekend. She sent a short disjointed text about being sick after her dad tried calling. This was followed by an awkward phone call several days later. Dan was experiencing déjà vu. For just a moment, he was 16 again listening to his mom talk on the phone telling him everything was fine. It was the tone in her voice. It sent chills through his body. Her words said one thing but the tone, pitch, and timing triggered something inside him. He knew, just like he knew with his mom. How could he have missed it with his daughter? That was the thought racing through his head that I was cheering on.

There it went again, the ringtone for her dad. Julie finally followed my suggestion to shut her phone off. She didn't need to be listening to her dad right now, she needed to be listening to me, and I was doing a lot of talking in her head. She had briefly entertained the idea of telling her parents about what her uncle had done to her, reasoning that it would take the heat off of her problems at school. I let her run through the presentation in her mind for an hour or two before I joined the conversation to point out the error of her reasoning. The whole Uncle John thing was a secret that needed to be kept. I only reveal secrets when it serves my purpose, and right now it didn't. First, I reminded her that she was a willing participant with Uncle John and what would her dad think of that? It would just crush him, and did she really want to hurt him like that? And then there was Adam, he would get into trouble because he kept the secret too. And what if they don't believe you? And with that thought we had lift off. Her anxiety and paranoia filled her dorm room like water in one of those disaster movies. She was out the door before I could start my next thought.

What most people don't understand about situations like Julie's is that it really isn't about getting high, buzzed, or stoned. She just wanted to not feel what she was currently feeling. And that's my specialty. I not only take the pain away, I take the feelings away. Lesson 1 - What causes pain? Feelings. Lesson 2 - How do we stop the pain? Stop the feelings. Julie was having a lot of feelings that she needed my help with. We were on a mission to quiet her anxiety. Her experience from two weeks ago of "blacking out" as you people call it still haunted her. I assured her it was just a fluke. She had been working hard at school and was run down. People forget stuff all the time and she really didn't need to worry. We decided, just to be safe, not to go back to the frat house. We'd swing by to visit a couple of upperclassman co-ed's we had met at a party at the beginning of the semester. I agreed to Julie's decision to limit our consumption to just two drinks. It seemed reasonable. I was just glad we had picked up the Alprazolam yesterday. Julie had visited the campus counseling center and they in turn referred her to the campus clinic where they gave her a script for Xanax. I convinced her now would be a good time to try one.

We slept great! And the dreams – well I guess that's a matter of perspective. Julie thought they were funny. There were these hot guys, music, this strange buzzing sound, and a tattoo place inside a fast food restaurant with a tiny little dog that kept licking her nose. It was all a bit bizarre as she thought about it. But whatever, she felt great. No anxiety and well rested. We slept in until almost noon. I was hungry, but Julie wanted to take a shower before we headed to the dining hall to get something to eat. She grabbed her robe and shower-basket and headed across the hall to the dorm bathrooms. She couldn't believe how good she felt, it was like she had a whole new outlook on life. The shower felt great. She put her wet hair up in a towel and wrapped her dripping body in her robe and headed back to her dorm room. Her roommate was gone for the weekend so she had the room to herself. She dropped her robe as she bent down to reach into her underwear drawer to get a bra and panties. When she glanced at the full length mirror that hung on the inside of her wardrobe door....well....you know how for you humans something doesn't hurt until you see it? I think some people call it a tramp stamp. There on her back, right at her panty line was this cute little red heart with wings – we both thought it was cute when we picked it out last night at that tat parlor next to the pet store. Apparently Julie didn't think it was cute anymore.

Cindy, Julie's mom, didn't buy into her husband's suspicion and paranoia about what might be going on with Julie. Dan's hyper-vigilance on the topic had been the focus of many arguments between them over the past few months. Cindy would drone on and on and on "Why can't you just trust her? Why do you think there always has to be something else going on? It's always something or someone with you! Blah-blah-blah." I liked Dan. He's been one of my loyal lemmings over the years serving me in a variety of support roles. He was my and his mommy's little helper, from a very early age. "Don't tell daddy" was one of his mom's favorite sayings. In a wonderful and unique way, it gave him a special purpose and a distinct bond between mother and son. It was something only the two of them shared, until he overheard her say it to his younger brother John. He could still remember exactly where he was standing in his parent's home when it happened. He was coming back from the kitchen with mommy's "medicine" just about to round the corner of the dark brown couch where she always laid when he heard her whisper to John, "This will be our little secret." He almost wet himself, he felt so betrayed. I think he was about 8 or 9 at the time. His parents still live in the same house.

The couch is gone, but he feels the pain of that moment every time he walks over that spot on the floor. He still hears it in his head, it triggers a ton of guilt and a storm of anger – I love it!

Dan and Cindy's arguments over whether Julie was in trouble had progressed to battles of extended silence. Sort of like one of those movies depicting World War I trench warfare where everyone just sits in their hole, except in Dan and Cindy's case, he sat at his desk and she curled up in their recliner. The vibration from his cell phone broke what had become a relatively comfortable silence. He scrambled for the phone to try and restore the silence – it was his mom. "Why isn't she calling John," he thought. "Why can't anyone in this family see that I have my hands full with Julie – no one in this family ever sees what is really happening," his thoughts continued. He pushed the screen to answer the call.

Dan's panic over Julie was overtaken by a medical thing with his brother John. John had been admitted to the hospital for chronic pancreatitis and liver issues. *This always happens to me in one fashion or another. My work is done on human canvases, and unfortunately for me, they don't last that long. John was hospitalized for 10 days. Two weeks after he was released from the hospital he was of no more use to me. I think John was weak and just gave up. His funeral could prove to be fertile ground for a few more of my conceptions. Julie's great, but I could see myself working with her brother Adam as well. While it may seem counter intuitive, once I've established a relationship with one member of the family it's really not that hard to extend my presence to more family members.*

When humans like John do give up, I get a lot of unfair bad press. Accusations of alcohol poisoning, too many drugs or scripts, too much this or that, are spread by anyone and everyone. It's a myth propagated to discredit me and sell news stories. People like Dr. Drew, Dr. Phil or Oprah are always spouting lies about me in an effort to promote themselves. When they're gone, another bunch of doctors and pundits will appear with new lies or reruns of the old ones. History's on my side. I've been helping humans escape your pain for as long as there's been humans. If what I do doesn't work, explain to me why the line at my door extends out of sight?

20

PETER & KAREN

By the time his mandated counseling was over, I don't know who was more frustrated, Peter or his youth pastor. Each week Peter's bitterness and resentment grew as a result of his discussions with the pastor. If he didn't want to use before he arrived at the mandatory meetings, he most definitely wanted to by the time he left, and he did.

Over the next eighteen months, I achieved my perfect mix of controlled chaos in Peter's family. I kept his parents in a state of emotional exhaustion and spiritual numbness – they had surrendered. His sister was busy packing on the pounds trying to make herself big enough to be noticed. And Peter, he was producing and maintaining the perfect level of stress and tension within the family to keep everyone playing their part. I believe the social work Nazis call it homeostasis – I call it home sweet home. Normal was now redefined according to my standards and resistance to my growth and development was at a manageable level.

Peter ended up with a minor in possession charge just weeks after he had finished being tortured by the pastor. He got a years' worth of juvenile probation. It was a minor speed bump in the scope of things and a great way to test his devotion to me. Peter quickly discovered Cannabicyclohexanol – it's harder to spell than marijuana, but it has its advantages – namely it doesn't show up on the standard THC drug screens. The IQ requirement to become a probation officer must be about three. Do you people really think you can outsmart or contain me? Your efforts are laughable at best. I've been around longer than any of you and I'm smarter than all of you – yet you still think you can stop me.

Karen had yet to meet a scale that she couldn't eventually break. As I've already said, food may not be the most glamorous of mediums to work with, but it does get the job done. She eventually broke the three hundred pound mark, which more than qualified her for gastric bypass surgery, which she underwent a couple of years prior to Peter

70

ceasing to be. You humans will go to such drastic lengths in your attempts to defeat me. Just because you mechanically disable your digestive system doesn't mean I'm going to loosen my grip on your brain. At best, all I'm going to do is readjust my grasp. Although I will admit, the first year after she did it, I think even I was starting to get depressed.

As always, I adjusted and adapted to the situation. But talk about an emotional black hole – if I hadn't stepped back in and helped her, I think she might have killed herself – kind of ironic if you think about it. Food could no longer produce the necessary shift in her neurotransmitter chemistry to provide the emotional regulation she craved. As much as she initially hated the idea, I knew alcohol was the best solution to her problem. Gastric bypass surgery produces the perfect hybrid for alcohol consumption. Whereas in the past, a person got twenty-five mpg relative to an alcohol buzz, after the physical modification to the stomach they'll get seventy-five - one-hundred mpg. A little goes a very long way, and it didn't take Karen long to figure that out.

21

JULIE

Julie dropped out of college in the middle of the first semester of her sophomore year. The demands of school simply was too much competition with our relationship. Do you like surprises? I do! I also like the word unbeknownst because it means there's a surprise just around the corner. Julie's parents, unbeknownst to them, were going to be grandparents. Actually that was unbeknownst to Julie as well, as she was too preoccupied with me to notice what else she had missed last month. The impregnation occurred during one of her blackouts just before her parents pulled her out of college. The father of this new grandchild is unbeknownst to everyone – technically there were four possible candidates from her last blackout. They better start studying for their paternity test – but I doubt any of them will ever be identified – Julie doesn't even know she had sex that night.

Julie was living at home, working part-time at the family grocery store. She hated that store. Over the past few months, when she wasn't in a blackout, she had been wrestling to understand how her special relationship with her Uncle John had begun. "How did it start? When did it start? Why didn't dad or mom protect me? Where were they when it happened?" "They were at the store, stupid!" OK that last thought was me not her, but she claimed it for her own. "They left you alone with a pedophile while they went to their precious store." That was me again.

She told her parents that there had been "some" use of alcohol while she was at school and that was all her dad needed to hear. He forced her to attend lame outpatient counseling as a condition of living at home. Each week the counselor would ask her about trauma and each week she would deny it. John had taken their secret to his grave. Julie was planning to do the same and had not told a soul about that part of her life – even though thinking of it was a regular part of almost each and every day. That one little secret was like a nuclear fuel rod that powered our relationship. It made everything so easy, almost boring. But like any love affair, the early part of the journey is always filled with excitement and anticipation – the end, not so much. But I had a feeling Julie and I were still going to have some exciting times.

Her brother Adam had moved to the other side of the state after getting married the previous year. He didn't know it yet, but his new wife's first love was actually me, not him. He was now acting as a caretaker for another one of my masterpieces in the making. He's going to be so mad when he finds out. I understand his frustration, having to serve me without any of the benefits, but he needs to accept his role for now – if I'm feeling benevolent in the future, I might offer him some relief. We'll see.

Julie had started to put on a few pounds even before she dropped out of college. She assumed it was because she had stopped her long distance running and was doing more stress related eating. While she had a few vague and confused memories related to a couple of sexual encounters during her freshman year, she had no memories of having sex during her short time at school the beginning of her sophomore year. She was becoming confused and concerned over her increasing size. She finally realized she had missed her period, but wasn't actually sure how many she had missed. Can you say insane? We were beginning to ponder that possibility. I knew she wasn't, but knowledge is power and I never relinquish my power. She was between your proverbial rock and a hard place. Can you imagine telling a doctor, or your parents for that matter, "I've missed my period, but I'm not sure how many I've missed, and my stomach is starting to look like I swallowed a volleyball, but I'm pretty certain I haven't had sex in over nine months, at least I don't remember having sex in the past nine months." But it's not a dream – you really can't fasten your jeans under that oversized shirt you're wearing!

Cindy got the call early on a Monday afternoon from one of the workers at the store. Julie had collapsed at work and was bleeding. The paramedics were at the store and were just getting ready to take her to the ER. Dan had been helping their son Adam and his new wife with a home remodeling project and was five hours away. Cindy tried to reach him on his cell but got his voice mail – she left a panicked message. As she drove to the ER, all kinds of scenarios ran through

73

her mind. Had she been on a ladder? Bleeding? Did the co-worker say she had fallen or that she collapsed? She couldn't remember. Her assumption was that she must have hit her head and that's what the bleeding was about. Just try to imagine her disconnect when the ER doc leads with, "Your daughter and her baby are fine." Who wants to break the news to grandpa?

Cindy was in shock, Julie was hysterical and had to be medically sedated – that was nice, and the ER doc was confused, suspicious, and had requested a psych eval. The doc estimated Julie was about eighteen weeks along. When Dan arrived and was told the news he was speechless for about five minutes and then he went straight to anger fueled by feelings of betrayal. "That little liar! She's been lying this entire time! She's just like my mom," was the thought that ran through his head – "they always lie about everything! Pregnant! She never mentioned she was even dating anyone. That lying little whore!" His thought, not mine.

One thing I like about humans is your incessant need to label everything, or more precisely everyone. Technically you're describing the behavior of the individual, but for some reason you pin it on the person as their identity; liar, whore, loser, addict, drunk, tweaker, bag bitch. Your list of derogatory descriptors is endless. When you run out of titles you either create new ones or you combine the old ones. I find them so useful. When you say them out loud I help your listener commit them to memory. When you don't verbalize them but communicate them with your eyes, I help your observer interpret the meaning of your condescending gaze, and commit that to memory. I sometimes prefer that form of communication because it allows me to be more creative and go into thesaurus mode with your observer and use a wider variety of identity labels to interpret your gaze.

Julie's collapse at the store was attributed to exhaustion and not enough calories in early pregnancy. She hadn't been eating the previous couple of weeks in an effort to fasten her jeans. Julie had actually felt some relief when she discovered the spotting as she thought her period had started. The heavy spotting concerned the ER doc and she put her on bed rest until Julie could follow up with an obstetrician.

She was released to go home after spending the entire night in the ER. Her mom had brought her home and she was resting in her bedroom. This was the same room where her brother Adam had walked in on her and Uncle John some seven years earlier. Her dad hadn't spoken to her since shortly after arriving at the hospital the previous evening. He was sitting at the kitchen table when Julie and her mom walked into the house. The look on her dad's face when their eyes met spoke volumes and cemented my relationship with Julie for years to come – not that our relationship was ever in question, but nonetheless, thanks dad!

Another of my superpowers that humans are unaware of is my ability for time travel – in either direction. I can take you into the future and show you how I can rescue you from all the pain inflicted by your family, your so called friends, your boss, or your co-workers. I can also transport you back in time to re-experience one of our first romantic encounters together and relive all the euphoric details. I've found that some humans, at least on a limited scale, also possess this power. In this case Julie's mom appeared to have transported herself back in time some fifteen years or so. She was singing this weird soft rhyming song about Julie's favorite blanket, as she was tucking the edges in around Julie's shoulders. Julie remembered the song and for a moment was transported back in time as well. That special blanket had been present during many of our special times with her now deceased Uncle John.

As Julie lay in her bed her thoughts bounced in several directions. There were her escapades with her Uncle John and her struggle to understand the origins of that relationship, her role in that relationship, and why her parents hadn't protected her. She had done so well in high school, but ended up being a total academic failure in college – what happened? Prior to college she had never experienced what she had considered a failure. Even though her brother Adam accidentally discovered her relationship with her uncle, other than that one episode, she had successfully kept their secret for six years. I always told her she should take pride in that accomplishment. And then there were all the vacant spots in her memory over the past twelve months. Tattoo's usually come with a story – she didn't have one. She *had lost bras and underwear after she had put them on – but didn't have a story for that either. She was pregnant but couldn't remember the conception. What would she tell her child on Father's Day?*

22

ANTON & SUSAN

The big celebration, by all surface accounts, went off without so much as a hitch. Anton, Susan, her parents, two other couples from their church, and a half dozen rug rats participated in celebrating my conception date – which also happened to be the anniversary of Anton killing the little girl on the twins' second birthday. It was an extra special day because the twins were now the same age as the girl their father had killed. I so wish you could've seen what was happening below the picture perfect surface. Susan and Anton had both doubled up on their Klonopin over the anticipation of the event. They didn't stop moving for a second during the party out of fear their thoughts would overrun them. Susan's parents were also having flashbacks behind their smiles. It was just two years earlier that they took care of the twins while Susan went to the ER to pick up their son-in-law.

The two other couples at the party could sense the uneasy tension but had no idea of its origin because they didn't know what we were really celebrating. Shortly after the killing, Anton and Susan left their church. It's a standard part of my strategy to isolate my prey. The isolation intensifies the loneliness and helps to slowly build the pain. It's an easy strategy with humans because you actually think it helps – you reason that if you don't have to talk about "it" or have to explain "it" then, "it" will be less painful. Most often you work with me in this strategy by humiliating your fellow humans. It all works so well. And then on top of all of this, when humans follow this strategy, then they have to live their lie. And that makes for exhausted humans.

The silence was deadening. The party was over. Anton was sitting in his favorite chair in their family room. He had fought all day to try to block out the image of Rachael in her last moments of life as she sat in the backseat of her parents' car. He had never spoken her name since he had heard it at the scene of the accident. The more he tried not to see her face, the more it appeared in his mind.

He could hear his breath as it moved in and out of his lungs. He was staring at the small clock that sat on the credenza. He thought he could see the minute hand moving. He had turned thirty a few months earlier. "My life sucks," was the repetitive thought that kept beating in his brain, interspersed with, "My life wasn't supposed to be like this." He hated Susan for abandoning him. Sure they were still together – but the nature of their relationship had changed – it was now a ménage à trois – a threesome - with me in the middle. And I don't like to share. It's just not part of my character.

Each of them had developed a monogamous relationship with me, leaving the other one out in the cold. Within a week or two after Susan had started to pilfer Anton's Klonopin, he was on to her. He was absolutely livid, but by that time, he was already doubling up on his own use of the script, so it made it a bit awkward for him to call her out on stealing his pills. I quickly pointed out to him that Susan must have a stash somewhere and all we needed to do was be patient and find it. And we eventually did. We then began to justifiably take back what had been stolen from us.

My ability to stay ahead of you humans is really quite impressive, if you're honest. From my throne room deep inside your brain, I nurture you with the motivation of hyper-vigilance. I start with simple confusion and suspicion. "I thought you had fifteen pills left? You better count them again. I know we had fifteen, count them again to make sure. What do you mean one's missing? There should be fifteen! If we didn't take it who did? Someone knows!" I then guide you into what I call practical paranoia. In the same way you can't steer a parked car, it's difficult to steer a non-paranoid human. By fostering just the right level of practical paranoia, I create the emotional movement and dance in humans that allows me to steer. Anton and Susan were now dancing with me, their pain, and their paranoia.

The Klonopin by itself wasn't doing it for Anton any longer, even when I had him doubling up on his pills. Tolerance is like gravity, it exerts a force of attraction that pulls humans into a deeper relationship with me. For Anton, it was time to deepen our relationship and augment our emotional pain management strategy. I debated my *options. Sex would be an easy option. Gambling's also easy and it fits well with sex, but each human reacts differently to that combination and sometimes they flame out in a very short time. It's fun to watch and it's usually a good ride, but generally short lived. I wanted a longer relationship with Anton.*

I like to be practical and use what's available. Susan had been a dual user since my birth and always preferred the sedation of an alcohol-benzo cocktail. Anton had never been drawn to alcohol, but I was sure I could win him over without much effort. A human's decision to accept the help I offer occurs when the pain they are experiencing has no apparent end in sight. And fortunately for me, most humans can't see very far. I began to echo Anton's repetitive thoughts in his head. "Your life sucks, it wasn't supposed to be like this." I threw in a few comparison shots across the bow. "Your friend Mike sure has a charmed life, he has all the toys you want but don't have, he has a super-hot wife, they just got back from Cabo San Lucas, they probably had sex on the beach, you've never had sex on the beach, the way things are going you'll probably never have sex again – your life REALLY sucks!" It works every time! Anton was up and headed for the kitchen – he needed something, he just wasn't sure what. He assumed the position in front of the open refrigerator scanning the shelves. Not to digress but I wonder - has anyone ever calculated how much time humans spend staring into their refrigerators? It's got to be a big percentage of your life. Anton locked on the orange juice just behind the bottle of red wine. He pulled out the wine bottle in order to reach the orange juice. "You need something different," I whispered. "Has orange juice ever helped you feel better?" I continued. To be technically correct, I probably should have said, "Has orange juice every stopped you from feeling your pain?"

Anton squeezed the cold glass neck of the wine bottle in his hand. It felt different – squeezing it felt good – it felt powerful, which was something he hadn't felt in a very long time. "We need different," I reminded him again. He let go of the refrigerator door and looked at the bottle as he cradled it in his other hand. "Susan will be pissed if I drink her wine," he thought to himself. It was more a statement of defiance than concern.

As we walked back to his chair in the family room with a large glass of wine I suggested we surf the net for some further distractions. Anton scanned his favorite news sites. Have you noticed that every major news outlet has an entertainment section? Like I said earlier, I use what's available. Let's see, the new SI swimsuit edition just came out with pics and video, there's a great article on the best celebrity beach bodies, and then there's always the latest celebrity sex tape that's making the news. I let Anton pick. Just four clicks later and Anton wasn't thinking about any of his problems or how much his life sucked.

This is what I call a neurological triple play. First add a benzodiazepine. Then add another sedative, in this case alcohol. And finally, take both of these in the context of sexual stimulation. What do these three things have in common? They all produce wonderful chemical responses in the limbic system of your brain – my home.

23

KAREN & PETER

Remember porky Karen? She was 28 when she attempted to leave me. She had that stomach plumbing surgery and got it in her head that she could remake her life and live without me. The lies you humans believe. Live without ME? Really? It's usually just a matter of hours, if not minutes, before you're running back to me begging for my help. You little creatures forget that I occupy the high ground in your brain called your limbic system – OK technically it's the low ground but that's beside the point! It's like holding your breath and telling yourself you're not going to breathe anymore. Go ahead and give it a try. When you wake up you'll be breathing and I'll still be here. You can't stop me, you can't wish me away, you can't wash me away, and you can't cast me out. I am. You, you are irrelevant. Without me there is no you! Karen would eventually learn that lesson.

She lost close to half her total body weight within the first year after the bypass surgery. I personally found that phase a bit irritating. She was too distracted by the whole process and wasn't focusing enough on our relationship – I knew she would eventually snap out of it and come back to me – all of you do. She was now, "attractive" for the first time in her life. According to those around her she had lost the weight in the, "right places" and her new curves had a magnetic quality that brought new interest from the males she would encounter. I could use this.

At the same time that her mass was shrinking, the number of orbiting males around her was increasing. And while all of this was happening, her brother Peter was about to become a supernova. Their dad kept threatening to throw fecal matter into a fan when it came to Peter – personally I don't get that metaphor, but his dad used it all the time. The groundless ultimatum appears to be a very common practice among humans. You use counting when attempting to get small humans to do what you want, "I'm going to count to three....one, two....two and half....." With big humans you make statements

23

predicting behavioral change on your part that are predicated upon the other person's future behavioral change, but then no one actually follows through on any of the predicted or predicated behavior. It's such a fascinating and meaningless human social protocol.

Peter and I were doing fine. He was now in his late 20's. His parents however, had way too much time on their hands and were attempting to pull together an intervention. That's a meeting where a bunch of you get together and tell vicious lies about me in an attempt to kill my human host by separating them from the life sustaining relationship they have with me. They got a couple of his so-called friends together, along with not-so-porky anymore Karen, and met with an interventionist to plan my demise. I knew what they had planned. Karen was my snitch. At the time, my relationship with Karen wasn't as healthy as it should have been, so I wasn't completely sure as to her motivation. I was hoping it was out of her loyalty to me, but then again she really hated her brother for ruining her teen years with all of his chaos. Maybe that's why she told him what they had planned. The intervention never took place – I made sure of that. However they did come to Peter's funeral a few months later after he ceased to be. No it wasn't me – I never cause anyone to cease. That happens as a result of their own stupidity. In Peter's case it was severe head trauma from not being coordinated enough to sit on the railing of a third floor apartment balcony. Ouch!

Karen's new-found sexuality - that had been hidden under 150 pounds of lard - was generating a wonderful emotional storm in her world. Combine that with all of the family drama around Peter's demise and we had the perfect level of anxiety to produce clarity of thought on her part – she still needed me. But we needed a new medium to work with due to the remodeling of her digestive system. And as I mentioned earlier, gastric bypass surgery produces the perfect hybrid for alcohol consumption. And take one guess what the modus operandi was for all those males that wanted to enjoy Karen's new and improved curves? Alcohol – the human fuel of choice in the race to copulate. Some things are just too easy.

24

JULIE

Do you have a best friend? Someone who will do anything to protect you? Stigma is my best friend. She leverages family, friends, and society, and is often my greatest protector. She is empowered by pride and prejudice. You, and those close to you, will construct elaborate stories because of her. She is my bodyguard, and like many of you, is willing to take a bullet for me. Julie's family had a new houseguest – my best friend, Stigma, was now living with them.

Cindy and Dan were in panic mode as they scrambled to create cover stories for all the drama. The phone was starting to ring and Facebook postings were flying in all directions with "concerned" inquiries. "Is Julie all right?" "What happened to Julie at the store yesterday?" "I heard Julie had to be taken to the ER, everything OK?" "Can we help with anything?" "Do you need anything?" Other helpful comments followed; "I'm sure she'll be fine with a little rest." "Whatever it is, she'll snap out of it." "This kind of thing happens to a lot of kids when they start college."

They decided to go with the storyline of stress and fatigue from over-exerting herself at college – everyone knew what a hard working over-achiever she was – it just all caught up with her when she went away to college. She just needed to take some time off and was going to be visiting some distant relatives in a neighboring state so she could rest up and collect her thoughts. That was the storyline. Dan, who had been more helpful to me when he was younger was now becoming a bit of a pain. He had located one of those treatment places for Julie to go and stay at until she had the baby. It was about seven hours away, not too far from where her brother Adam and new wife Rachel were living.

I kept assuring Julie we would be fine, we just needed to go with the flow for a couple of months, say what they all wanted to hear, and eventually we could put some distance between us, her parents, and everyone else that wanted to separate us. Julie had stopped her use of alcohol because of the pregnancy and was relying on her Xanax script to meet my needs. We both felt a bit of panic when her parents told her the place they were sending us wouldn't allow our Xanax. I can hold my breath for quite a while and I knew they wouldn't be able to keep us there forever.

The seven hour ride to our new home was mind numbing even for me. It was just the four of us in the car and no one spoke except her mom. She just kept looking at the brochure and reading sections of it to us. "I'm sure you'll enjoy it once you get settled into a routine, look they have a workout room and a sauna. It says here they have therapeutic dogs that visit each week. And there's a nutritionist that plans the meals. Look at that beautiful dining room. I think you're really going to like it here." We stopped for gas around hour three. Julie and I went to the restroom – it was the only way we could get a moment alone. Julie was contemplating what it might be like to just stay in the restroom for the rest of her life. I assured her everything would be OK, she just needed to keep trusting me – I'd take care of her, I always had.

Hour five had us stopping by her brother and sister-in-law's place. Julie had only seen Adam and Rachel once since they got married in the fall of her freshman year. I love these awkward gatherings. Julie and I were pondering the possible conversations as we walked up to the apartment building with her parents, "So...how was school?" " I flunked out....I've been working at the store." "That must suck. Looking forward to treatment?" "Sure, can't wait!" The actual small talk was different, but nonetheless awkward. Julie and I made a strategic retreat to the bathroom. She could hear them talking in the other room. "How long will she be there? When is she due, will she have the baby there? Is she going to keep it? Where's the father? Blah, blah, blah." Julie stopped paying attention. She didn't have to pee, she just wanted to escape. I suggested we explore the medicine cabinet, as I'm always looking for opportunities. There was something about Rachel that resonated with Julie. They had only been in the room together for about five minutes, but Julie could see it in her eyes. Julie didn't know what "it" was, but they definitely had a connection...which happened to be me. And there it was on the top shelf in the back, right corner, vitamin K, or as you call it, Klonopin. Xanax and Klonopin are basically cousins. The Klonopin wasn't going to kick in as fast as the Xanax, but it would eventually help calm our fears, and it would last longer.

Despite her poor academic performance in college, Julie was actually very intelligent. Not that it matters all that much to me, but having an intelligent host does have its advantages. All of that brain power and ingenuity is at my disposal. The script had just been recently refilled and was almost full. Julie quickly searched the other bottles to see if there was anything that resembled the size and color of Klonopin. She found something close and swapped out twenty of the Klonopin with the substitutes and mixed them in with the bottom half of the bottle. She thought for a moment and then quickly removed her tennis shoes. She pulled out the inserts and tore out part of the foam to make a small cavity in each. She split the twenty Klonopin, wrapped them in toilet paper and hid ten in each shoe and slipped them back on her feet. "Are you OK in there?" Her mom was at the door. "Yup, just a little nauseous." Julie flushed the empty toilet and opened the bathroom door. After a bit more awkward conversation, we were back in the car on the final leg of our journey – but feeling a whole lot more at peace.

It was late afternoon when we arrived. Our new home was located in the middle of nowhere. Cow pastures and corn fields for as far as the eye could see. There were about a dozen buildings of various sizes spread over about ten acres. It reminded me of the old television show Little House on the Prairie, but with more corn and slightly upgraded buildings. The closest major city was about fifteen miles away. The founders had theorized that the captives held at the facility wouldn't be able to walk away in such a rural area. Never underestimate my followers. There was a truck stop six miles away by road, but only about a mile through the corn field. They sold alcohol. You simply jumped the small, white decorative fence behind the maintenance building, counted twenty-one rows of corn from the corner of the building, and walked down that row for about a mile and you would come out right behind the truck stop. It's a little tricky in the dark, but my followers were committed.

Julie had about fifteen minutes with her parents before they had to leave, so she could begin her indoctrination. They wouldn't be back for two weeks - that was the first time family members would come back to visit someone new to the torture process. The torture began with peeing in a cup! They made us do it while her parents were still there just in case we failed their test. I must have dozed off while we were sailing through the sea of cornfields. If I wouldn't have been sleeping, I would have convinced Julie to take one of those Klonopin in her shoes, then we could have failed the test and drove home. We tried using tears to get her parents to take us back home, but it didn't work. I always had told Julie her parents were cold and uncaring individuals, this just proved me right again. Unfortunately, the Klonopin were discovered in the baggage and clothing search and were confiscated. They ended up in a mixture of kitty litter goo. They say it's the safest environmental way to dispose of pharmaceuticals. I think they do it that way just to try and humiliate me. It doesn't work.

25

KAREN

It seemed so real. Peter was there sitting on the edge of the balcony smiling. Karen wanted to pull him back from the edge and was trying to reach him but she couldn't move. Peter just leaned back and disappeared over the edge. It was 3:00 am and her nightgown was soaked with sweat. It was just like the night before. The dream haunted her. The guilt over her brother's death and their contentious teen years was crushing her soul. That's how she explained it to the counselor she was seeing. The last time she spoke to Peter she had given him her standard speech about what a loser he was, and how he had made their lives a living hell growing up. She hated all the attention he got from their parents. What she really hated was the lack of attention directed at her. I don't think she actually wanted him to die. Either way, I was there to help and comfort her.

For the first time in her life, I actually had competition. There were a lot of guys that wanted to comfort her too. Curves are curves, and Karen had a lot of them when she lost three hundred plus pounds. But she discovered something when she got down to one hundred and thirty pounds. She discovered she had power. Power to attract and manipulate men. She loved it. It was intoxicating. Unfortunately for Karen, the men discovered something as well. Get one drink into Karen and they would have full access to all the right places. I won't bore you with all the technical details, but when you bypass the stomach, the alcohol you drink goes straight into your large intestines and gets absorbed almost immediately. My favorite word.

Jim and Nancy felt like they had been transported back in time when they got the call that Karen was at the ER. Peter had ceased to be from his fall before they were able to get to the ER. History didn't repeat itself this time. Karen continued to live, but just barely. She had been at a bar playing a drinking game with friends from work. I guess it depends upon your point-of-view as to how you define winning the game, but Karen definitely excelled at alcohol absorption.

She went unconscious after five quick drinks. The loss of consciousness was actually from absorbing the alcohol from the first two drinks. The other three were still being absorbed in her intestines after she passed out, while they waited for EMS to arrive. The fourth one sedated her brain to the point of respiratory arrest. That breathing thing is important, and Karen was just lucky someone noticed she wasn't.

The ER was the usual chaotic mix of panic, tears, and anger, all the normal family stuff. In addition to her parents, her younger brother Jake was there, as well as her older brother Dan and his wife. Jake just kept holding her hand while the others argued over what needed to happen next. It was odd that the one person who was considered handicapped or special needs was doing more for Karen than the other four combined. He just held her hand. Karen had been out of her parents home for several years, and they had no idea of the depth of her devotion to me. There's usually a direct relationship between your level of devotion and the amount of pain I've relieved. Even though I've seen it countless times, I'm always fascinated that humans, even in the context of families, can't see the pain of others. You only feel your own. That's why it's so easy for me to divide and conquer. There's very little dividing that has to be done because you do it for me. And most of the time, I simply claim you rather than conquer you.

Karen only stayed in the hospital for one night. She spent the next week at her parents home. Dan stopped in a couple of times to visit her. He was six years older than Karen and had left the house for college by the time all the drama with Peter had started. He and Karen never really connected because of the age difference. Jake still lived at home with his parents and never left Karen's side during that week. When she was a teen, and having to watch all the attention Peter got, it would drive her crazy. Jake would want to follow her around. It was different now. She was actually enjoying Jake's company.

26

ANTON & SUSAN

Susan and Anton maintained the status quo for the next nine months. They both continued to serve me and provide for my needs quite well. And they did it with passion. At times even coming to blows over me. Having someone willing to fight over you just makes you feel truly cherished. It wasn't like an actual boxing match like you see on TV. It was more like a very physical dance. Susan would push and slap Anton, and Anton in turn would punch the wall. Of course the whole dance was done to a sound track of expletives. I know what you're thinking. Didn't they have a set of twins? Where were their twin girls when all this was going on? Daniel and Chanel were in the bedroom listening, usually with their covers over their heads. When it got really loud, they would get into bed together and hide under their pillows to try and stop the sound.

I really do try to help my people keep things going in the right direction for as long as possible. I liken myself to a surfer when they get on a good wave and want to ride it to the very end. I like to enjoy the ride and have fun, but sometimes humans are just so unpredictable. Susan was starting to get that way. Personally I like paranoia. A little hyper vigilance is a useful tool for me. But Susan was getting almost too unpredictable even for me, and that's saying a lot. It was a Saturday afternoon and Susan and Anton had been engaged in some moderate verbal exchanges for most of the day. Susan's mind was starting race. I was even having trouble keeping up. We both agreed it was probably time to tap into her new stash of Xanax.

She had secured a dozen of them about three weeks earlier at a community lunch presentation for some local cause. One of her friends had dragged her there against her will, but she felt obligated to attend. It was at the Marriott, in one of their mid-sized ballrooms, crammed with about forty round tables. Susan and her friend ended up at a table with seven other ladies they had never met. After what seemed like an eternity, their table had finally been sent to the buffet line. Susan managed to make it back to the table first. The woman who had sat next to her had left her purse on her chair. Susan happened to glance at it and instantly saw the telltale green of a script bottle peering through the narrow opening of the bag. She glanced back at the buffet line. She guessed she had between 45-60 seconds before anyone else returned. She was well practiced by now, and as soon as she saw the magic word Alprazolam, she knew she had gold. She had skimmed off about a quarter of the bottle and returned it to the bag within a matter of seconds. Lunch wasn't so bad after all.

She had hidden this new stash in the basement with the Christmas decorations. They were inside one of the large ornament balls. Susan pulled off the metal spring top from the ornament and held it on its side and gently shook the ball. Three of the pills slid into her palm. She carefully put one back into the decoration, and while holding the other two in her hand, she secured the metal cap back onto the ball and placed it back in the box. All the previous Xanax she had acquired were white but these were blue. Susan figured it was just a different manufacture. The racing thoughts continued to spin in her head. The thoughts were all her own, I didn't need to help. Her chest felt like she had a belt around it that had been pulled too tight. It hurt to breathe. She went into the bathroom in the basement and washed the two pills down with a handful of water from the sink. She had taken two of the Xanax before. There was only one small problem this time. It was her math. In the past when she had taken two, they were the white Xanax, which were .25 milligrams. Blue wasn't a different manufacturer, it was a larger dose! They were one milligram pills. Susan had taken four times her usual amount!

Susan returned to the kitchen to start dinner. Anton had opened a bottle of wine and poured himself a glass. He didn't offer, she helped herself. The first glass of wine always slowed things down. Even the twins, who were almost six now, could predict the storm. The calm was like the eye of the hurricane. It felt good, but you knew what was coming. They normally wouldn't get to the point of pushing, slapping, and wall punching until after the twins were in bed - it was still too early for that. Their home had an open kitchen where the dining area was just on the other side of a large island for food prep. The girls were at the table working on a jigsaw puzzle. Anton was getting the meat out of the refrigerator, and Susan was cutting carrots at the island. The glass of wine mixed with two milligrams of Xanax was new territory for Susan. She quickly began to feel warm. It was like her mind had been disconnected from her body. Her ability to cut the carrots was simply a body memory. She had done it so many times, she didn't need her brain to do it. Communication skills, however, required the brain to be awake. The alcohol combined with 8-Chloro-1-methyl-6-phenyl-4H-s-triazolo benzodiazepine made it almost impossible for Susan to receive or send any meaningful verbal messages.

She had no idea how much time had passed. She was still at the island with the carrots. She was only registering about every fourth or fifth word Anton was saying. He had confronted her about stealing pills from her friends. She just stared at him. When he walked over to the table and grabbed her purse from the chair and started opening it she chased after him and tried to grab it from him. She was sure the pills she took three weeks ago were still in the purse. She reached for the purse - the only problem was she still had the knife in her hand. I think the twins both screamed first, then Anton, Susan just stared speechless at the paring knife sticking in Anton's arm. The whole scene gave new meaning to family bonding around the dinner table. Susan and Anton were both intoxicated, so they wouldn't remember the scene in great detail. The twins weren't going to have that luxury.

Anton went to the ER by himself. He called a friend of Susan's to come over and watch her and the twins. Susan was almost catatonic. Anton thought he had put together a pretty good story about how the stab wound in his arm was an accident. It was a good story. Unfortunately standard protocol in the ER for a stab wound includes notifying the police. They showed up to discuss the evenings events with catatonic Susan while Anton was still at the hospital. There was also another little problem. Anton was legally intoxicated when he drove himself to the ER. So with one intoxicated father with a stab wound, and one intoxicated catatonic mother, Daniel and Chanel got to spend the night with their Child Protective Services emergency *foster care parents. I was the only one that had a good evening that night.*

AND I LIVED HAPPILY EVER AFTER

Do you want me to go on? I think I'm done now. I've probably told you more than I should, but I love my stories. It's not about John and Julie or Peter and Karen or any of the other humans I've mentioned. It's about me. There are a select few out there that know of my secret ways. They know how I hijack your neural pathway, separate you from your spirituality, and isolate you from family and friends. But those that know my true ways are few, and the vast majority of you don't believe them. You believe people have a choice when it comes to my domination. If they would just try harder maybe they could live without me. It's true you have some choices very early in our journey, but once I seize control of your soul and the key areas of your brain, you lose your choice, and you lose control, it's gone, you're mine.

So, let me tie up the loose ends for you.

John *~ After a good, long relationship with me, he ceased to be.*

Karen *~ After the week at her parent's home, Karen finally went back to her own place. Unfortunately, she continued to meet with her counselor for several months. I can only imagine that water boarding feels similar to the weekly sessions we had with her counselor. She was given the usual spiel and propaganda about how I was bad for her and that the only reason she was sick was because of me. It was the same old stuff, nothing original. With Karen, I think I finally got to the point where I just wasn't interested in her any longer. She was really starting to bore me. No excitement. No challenge. I just didn't have time for her any longer. I'm not sure what happened to her.*

Peter *~ Eventually, people cease to be. Peter did so earlier than most.*

Anton & Susan *~ My power couple. Now they're just power individuals. They stopped being a couple about two years after the cutting of the carrots got out of hand. They were never dull. Before* *they split up, Anton managed to run over Susan with his car. She was going to stop him from leaving by laying down in the driveway. It didn't work. But not to be out done, nine months later Susan broke half of the fourteen bones in Anton's face. With a frying pan.*

The twins, Daniel and Channel, became frequent flyers in the foster care system. They both know of me. Soon they'll know me.

Julie ~ *Julie quickly settled into the routine of the Little House on the Prairie, as I liked to call it. Her pregnancy went full-term and, she gave birth to a son about three months after arriving at the facility. It was about a month into her brainwashing when I really started to lose interest in her. She lacked the commitment of her Uncle John. John was willing to give me everything. Julie wasn't willing to surrender herself the way I needed her to. She just wasn't worth my time anymore, not when there were so many other deserving humans begging for my help.*

As I said when I began my story, I'm counting on you to keep my secrets – and you will. The bizarre insanity of my secrets creates its own unique camouflage. Even if you share what I've told you, few will believe you, and those that might, won't have a clue what to say or how to help. If it hasn't become clear yet, each one of you has a role and a part in my story – and for that I thank you. How does my story end? Seriously? My story doesn't end! I'm eternal. I've been here since man's first breath, and I will be here until your last. You need me. You couldn't survive without me.

I know what you're thinking, that should be apparent by now. Some of you are thinking, "This is whacked, I don't know anyone who's had the experiences described in this diatribe." You just keep right on thinking that.

The rest of you are wondering....how did I know?

PART 2
THE DIALOGUE
THE SOLUTION TO ADDICTION

A DIALOGUE - THE SOLUTION TO ADDICTION
(WITHOUT THE VOICE OF ADDICTION)

"If we don't start a dialogue, the monologue will continue."

I think we've all heard enough from addiction. The remainder of this book is about finding a path out of addiction. We will look at that path from two perspectives. The first perspective will be for anyone reading this that knows the voice of addiction all too well, because they are caught in its grip. The second perspective will be for those that have a friend or loved one struggling with addiction. If you happen to be in the second group with a loved one or friend that is struggling, be sure to read Perspective #1, please don't skip it. The same holds true if you're in group one, everyone needs to read and see both perspectives. They each have valuable information and insights that could help you.

PERSPECTIVE #1
I RECOGNIZE MYSELF IN THE ADDICTION MONOLOGUES

What do I do if I recognize myself as one of the characters in the Addiction Monologues? Short answer, you seek help. Probably not the solution you were hoping to hear. But I'm not going to lie to you because your life depends upon knowing how to free yourself from addiction. Freedom from addiction is found in deep inner healing, which is a journey and not a quick fix. I'll talk more later about how and where to ask for help.

In its most basic form, addiction arises out of our desire to escape the pain of our wounds. Many treatment programs and support programs focus on the symptoms of addiction (drug and alcohol use, gambling, sex, binge eating, etc.) and not the trauma and wounds that serve as the catalyst or source for creating the addiction. It is true that the symptoms of our particular addiction have to be addressed, with the desired outcome of remission, which means no active symptoms. But you cannot stop there. That is not healing. When it comes to addiction, getting rid of the symptoms (drinking, smoking, shooting, pill eating) is not healing. It is simply the absence of active symptoms. The physical craving, the thoughts of using, and the pain from trauma and other wounds, are all still present within us, under the surface.

*Several years ago, I underwent surgery to donate a kidney. I treated the post-op pain from my incision with a therapeutic dose of Tylenol. The Tylenol would - "make my pain go away" - for about five hours. This pattern continued for several days because the Tylenol wasn't healing the wound of my incision. My pain would continue until the wound of my incision healed. If the **source** of our pain - our wound - is not healed, the pain will return, and shortly after that, we will need to find a way to make our pain go away, again. The solution to pain is not to mask the pain, the solution to pain is to heal the wound that is responsible for it.*

I'm going to repeat my last statement because it is so important for us to know, understand, and accept; **The solution to pain is not to mask the pain, the solution to pain is to heal the wound that is responsible for it.** *Our journey to freedom begins by admitting to ourselves, and someone else, that the pain exists. We may not be able to pinpoint the exact source of our pain or explain it to others, but we must not deny that it is present and very real. The very next thing to do after admitting and recognizing our pain is to reach out and ask for help. This is important. Don't stop asking until you get the help you need.*

To get the help you need, you cannot hold back. You have to be completely honest. Sometimes we don't share information because no one specifically asks us a question about it. If you want to obtain freedom from addiction by healing the source of your pain, you must be honest and share everything you are aware of regarding the pain you feel along with your wounds.

Let me illustrate this with a story similar to the experience of Julie and Peter in the Monologue. I've heard this story way too many times. A woman, we'll call her Sarah, came to me about six months after completing a residential treatment program. Sarah, who was twenty-six, had relapsed just a few days earlier. Her drug of choice was alcohol and she had starting drinking again and wanted help to stop. I had not worked with Sarah in a treatment relationship, but I was aware that she had completed a treatment program earlier in the year. I asked her if she had any insights into why she had returned to drinking. She responded, "I've been wondering about that, and I really think it has something to do with the pain of being raped at age fourteen." I replied, "That makes sense. When you were at treatment did you talk with your therapist about the rape?" Sarah answered, "No, it never occurred to me that the two might be connected. I think they asked if I had ever been assaulted, but I didn't want to talk about it with them, so I answered no."

I can understand Sarah not wanting to talk about the rape. There will be parts of the healing journey that will be difficult, but necessary if we want to experience healing and freedom. Revealing our wounds is not something we should do with just anyone. You will want to connect with a trained and experienced professional. Someone that has specific training in both substance use disorders, addiction, AND trauma treatment.

ASKING FOR HELP

If you are a member of the Perspective #1 group, the fact that you are even considering asking for help puts you in an elite group. Statistics are not an exact science, but most researches estimate well over 90% of people in the Perspective #1 group never ask for any help. I'm glad you're here reading this. Keep reading.

For many of us, we don't ask for help because we don't trust the people around us. Often that is the voice of addiction. But it can also be the voice of experience, and in part due to the fact that addiction (our addiction) has taught those around us not to trust us. When you add to the mix the fact that very few people in our society really understand the complexity of addiction, it makes it difficult to overcome our fear of asking for help. But hear me, asking for help is worth it! It will start you on your journey of healing. The voice in our head screams, "No one will understand!" And that voice in your head may be correct. The first person you ask for help may not understand. But if you've reached out to someone who loves you and or cares about you, they may not understand, but they will still help you connect with people that do understand and can help you. Perspective #2 people - did you catch that? You don't have to understand it to help someone you love and care about connect with the help they need to get well.

Asking for help doesn't mean you have to be prepared or expected to share every ugly and painful detail of your struggle. Asking for help is about getting connected with the right people that can help us begin to heal. After we ask for help and get connected with the right person or group of people, there will be plenty of time to share the hard facts and trauma's of our journey that need healing. Let it unfold.

There are at least five common paths for seeking help:

1. *Asking a friend*
2. *Asking a family member*
3. *Asking your employer*

4. *Walking into a support group such as Alcoholics Anonymous (AA), Narcotics Anonymous (NA), Celebrate Recovery (CR) or SMART (Self Management and Recovery Training)*
5. *Directly contacting a professional treatment facility.*

I will explain each of these paths in slightly more detail, and I will also give you some idea of what to ask for in each situation.

ASKING A FRIEND OR ACQUAINTANCE

Friends come in all shapes and sizes. We have close friends and not so close friends (acquaintances). A friend could be a co-worker, a neighbor, someone we see each week at the gym, someone who attends our church, or someone we went to school with. It doesn't matter where they are or whether they are close or not so close. What matters is that you feel a level of trust in the relationship. Trust that they are the type of person that would offer to help you connect with the resources you need.

One day while I was working as an addiction therapist, two women walked into our agency lobby. The older of the two, who appeared to be in her mid forties, asked if they could speak with someone about getting help. I invited them back into my office. The older spokeswoman proceeded to introduce me to her younger friend, who was in her late twenties. The two of them had been working together for about two months. Earlier that day, the young woman had shared with her co-worker friend that she was struggling with drinking too much and wanted to get help. Her friend did a quick search of the internet for local resources, found the agency I was with, and then offered to not only drive the younger woman to our office, but to come in with her and stay with her through the intake and assessment process! WOW! I was blown away by this woman's kindness and willingness to help someone who she had only known for two months. The combination of what the two of them did that day, asking for help, and actually helping, may very well have saved this young woman's life! It's estimated that 88,000 people die from alcohol-related causes annually, which makes alcohol the third leading preventable cause of death in the United States. Our neighborhoods and workplaces need more people like her! Perspective #2 people - I hope this story, which is true, inspires you.

Potential phrases to start a conversation asking for help:

> *"Could I ask you a personal favor? I've been struggling with some things and I want to find someone that might be able to help. Do you know or have any ideas on who I might call or go see?"*

> *"Would you be willing to help me with something? I'm trying to find someone that I could talk with about some personal things that I've been struggling with."*

> *"Could I ask you question? Do you know anyone who's ever struggled with alcohol or something else like that and if they went anywhere to get help? I'm trying to find some resources."*

ASKING A FAMILY MEMBER

Family members also come in all shapes and sizes. We have close family members and sometimes we have family members that are shame machines for our addiction. Choose wisely, but know that just because a family member may have a tendency to shame us, doesn't mean they won't help. Shame is a hurtful tool misguided family members often use because they've never learned any other way. Check out the article, **Shame: The approach that keeps producing exactly what you don't want.** It's found in the 'More Resources' section at the end of the book.

When asking a family member for help, it's going to be important to stay on topic. The topic is asking for help. Don't allow yourself to be pulled into past arguments or new arguments. If your family member brings up the past or begins to shame you, it is up to you to redirect them to the question at hand - will they assist you in finding the help you need right now? If your family member, like a pit bull that lives in my house, likes to lock onto an argument and never let go of it, you need to simply and quickly let go and remove yourself from the conversation (argument), and find another person to ask.

Perspective #2 people - I hope you're reading this like I asked you to. Remember Addiction's strategy from the monologue? "It's a standard part of my strategy to isolate my prey. The isolation intensifies the loneliness and helps to slowly build the pain. It's an easy strategy with humans because you actually think it helps – you reason that if you don't have to talk about "it" or have to explain "it" then, "it" will be less painful. Most often you work with me in this strategy by humiliating your fellow humans. It all works so well." I write this with all sincerity, addiction doesn't need any help, especially from you. Your loved one needs your help and they are asking you for it. Help your loved one, don't help Addiction. Remember Karen in the monologues? She wanted to share her *struggle with her parents, but they didn't have time to listen. Perspective #2 people, please have time and listen without judgment or shame.*

How you approach your family will depend upon whether your family is aware of your struggle with addiction and how that struggle has been experienced in your family. If your family has little to no awareness of your struggle, they may have a wide variety of reactions. Disbelief is one possible reaction. Disbelief might result in them minimizing what you tell them. They might take the position that, "you really don't need that kind of help." In your moment of clarity, you KNOW that you do need that kind of help, don't accept your families disbelief. Another possible reaction is shock. Another might be anger. There will be a reaction when you ask for help. Remember to stay focused on the task at hand, which is getting the help you need.

If you think your family is largely unaware of your struggle, here's one approach you might want to consider:

> *"Could I ask you a serious question? If I needed help with something that may not make sense to you right now, would you still be willing to help me? I've been dealing with some stuff that I've never really talked about and I think I need to find someone - like a professional - to talk with and try and sort some things out.*

If your family is aware of your struggle, you can take a more direct approach. Take a moment and think about how you would like them to help you. If they've been aware of your struggle, they may already know of some resources that could be available to you. Your approach may be as straight forward as:

> *"It's time, I've been reading this book, and it's time for me to get some help. Would you help figure out how to do this?"*

If you've had some stumbles in your past attempts to get well, you will want to acknowledge those when you approach your family members:

> *"It's time, I've been reading this book and I've really learned some things about myself and about my struggle, I know in the past you've tried to help me and it didn't go well and I fought you on it. I really do want help and I'm trying my best to accept it."*

ASKING YOUR EMPLOYER

The thought of talking with your boss about struggling with addiction may have just shot your anxiety through the top of your head. Your reaction to that idea will depend upon your perception of your employer. The reaction of your employer will depend upon their perception of addiction and different mental heath struggles. We hope their reaction will be supportive of your getting help. Exactly how much support they can provide to you will be determined in part by the size of the business and the company's human resource policies. Some companies may provide you with a leave of absence while you get help and hold your job for you. The Family and Medical Leave Act (FMLA) provides employees with up to twelve weeks of unpaid, job-protected leave per year for certain medical reasons.

But I need to be clear, the number one goal is not holding onto your job. The number one goal is getting the help you need to save your life and get healthy. Keeping your job, if you still have it, is nice, but it's not the most important thing at this point in your journey. If you are currently holding a job, and place a higher priority on keeping your job than on getting the help you need, you will eventually lose both.

There are two possible options to consider when asking for help from your employer. If the company you work for is large enough to have a human resources department (HR) you could start there. If you have what you consider to be a good and supportive relationship with your supervisor you might want to start with them.

Here's one possible way to start the conversation:

> *"I've heard that I can apply for a program to get some time off to address a medical issue, is that true? Could you help me with the paper work or do you know someone that could? Could I ask you a*

107

couple of questions about the Family and Medical Leave Act? "

WALKING INTO A SUPPORT GROUP

While support groups are often the brunt of humor in movies, they have actually saved a lot of lives and they are not a bad place to start. There could be a variety of support group options depending upon where you live. Options might include:

- *AA - Alcoholics Anonymous*
- *NA - Narcotics Anonymous*
- *CR - Celebrate Recovery*
- *SMART - Self-Management and Recovery Training.*

One of the first things to consider is whether you know anyone, friend, family member, or co-worker that attends one of these groups? The groups all practice anonymity, not revealing the names of other people who attend, but many people are open about their own attendance at one of these groups. If you are aware of someone that attends one of these groups, you could approach them for more information.

"The other day I heard you mention a group you attend....is it helpful? I'm curious how you got connected with it, would you be willing to share a bit more with me? I'd like to learn more about it."

And then there is always our friend Google. A simple search of the phrase "Find an AA meeting" will probably produce over 150 million options for you. Start by looking at the top five or six. I just made that search, and I found a meeting fourteen minutes away from the couch I'm sitting on right now.

In most groups the question will be asked, "Are there any first time visitors here?" No need to fear, just remember that every single person in the room was at one time a first time visitor. Sit back and take it all in.

Now what? Maybe you want to come back to that meeting, maybe not. The first meeting you visit may not resonate with you, you may not feel the connection you were hoping for or expecting. That's okay. There's probably a few more meeting options on that list from Google. The best advice I've heard about meetings is to try out (visit) at least five before you decide if you want to connect with a certain group. It's like trying on new shoes, you want to make sure you find a good fit.

I want to encourage you to not limit your pursuit of help and healing to only connecting with a support group. Support groups can play a vital role in your getting well, but they work even better when you combine them with some form of professional treatment help.

CONTACTING A TREATMENT FACILITY

Let me say this upfront, my purpose is to reduce some of your anxiety about this step. For many people, this sounds and feels very scary. I understand that. But do you know what lies just beyond your fear? Your freedom. Everything we've been talking about up to this point is about getting you started on a new leg of your journey. This is about starting to live a new lifestyle. A lifestyle of being healthy and balanced. Professional treatment and coaching can help you start and maintain that new, balanced, healthy life. The next couple of paragraphs can feel very heavy and overwhelming. This is where you could ask a friend, family member, or coworker for help. They could help you navigate through this information to find the right resource for you.

If you have insurance, you can start by calling some of the numbers on the back of your insurance card. There should be a number for benefits and eligibility and there might also be a number for mental health and substance abuse preauthorization. It will depend upon your particular insurance, but there's always a number you can call on the back of the card and you can ask about participating providers in your area.

If you do your Google search, which I recommend, you will find a wide variety of options for professional treatment. There are a lot of opportunities for finding and connecting with the help that's just right for you! If you have a friend or family member that is supporting you in your decision to find help, you might ask them to help you contact and sort through some of your options. Here are some things to look for or ask about as you consider your options:

Is the treatment facility accredited? *Accreditation is similar to a personal reference. It means another organization has throughly examined or checked out the facility and vouches for them. The Commission on Accreditation of Rehabilitation Facilities (CARF)* and the _Joint Commission_, formerly known as JCAHO are two of the more common accreditation's.

Is the facility licensed by the state? _While licensing doesn't guarantee the quality of treatment, it does point to a higher level of professionalism and accountability._

What is the level of training for your staff? _You are looking for a professionally trained staff with a combination of experience and expertise. The therapists and counselors should have advanced training in the area of addictions. To be a Certified Advanced Alcohol and Drug Counselor (CAADC) you must have a master's degree and over two thousand hours of experience and specialized training in the treatment of addictions. An addictionologist is a medical doctor, often an anesthesiologist, that has an additional medical board certification for the treatment of addictions. Not every treatment facility will have an addictionologist on staff, but many facilities have a consultation relationship with an addictionologist. Some facilities may also have recovery coaches on staff to assist in the treatment process. Recovery coaches are individuals that have been in successful, sustained recovery for over a year and have specialized training to support those in treatment and early recovery._

Are you affiliated with any religious organizations, faiths, or church? _This is not necessarily a positive or negative. It is simply important for you to know and be aware of the philosophical perspective of the organization you are connecting with. While many treatment facilities rightly recognize the spiritual component of addiction and the need to address this component in the treatment and healing process, not all religious and faith based programs recognize the neurobiological aspects of addition that must be addressed for successful treatment._

The organization Narconon markets itself as a form of addiction treatment. Narconon has strong affiliations with the Church of Scientology. Many addiction treatment professionals would disagree with Narconon's statement that they provide addiction treatment.

Do you provide both detoxification services and treatment services? _That's a new big word - detoxification. What does it mean? Detoxification, in this context, is the process your body goes through_

112

to eliminate all of the particular substance you have been putting into your body. This process at times can be very uncomfortable/painful - we call it withdrawals. If your substance has been alcohol, from the point of your last drink it will take between thirty-six to seventy-two hours for all of the alcohol to completely leave your body. Because of the unique way alcohol works in our brain, if we've been using a lot of it, we might be at risk of having a seizure as the alcohol leaves our body. A good treatment facility will actually ask you questions about this during your initial phone screening to determine your most immediate need and whether you should receive detoxification services before treatment services. Not all treatment facilities provide detoxification services and not all detoxification facilities provide treatment services, and some provide both. Detoxification is not treatment, it is part of the process of stabilization before you start treatment. If you have ever had a seizure in your life, especially in the context of alcohol, you should go through a medically supervised detoxification before beginning formal treatment services.

Using the questions above should help you narrow down your choices and locate a good treatment facility. Another option to help in your search is SAMHSA's National Helpline – 1-800-662-HELP (4357). SAMHSA's National Helpline is a free, confidential, 24/7, 365-day-a-year treatment referral and information service (in English and Spanish) for individuals and families facing mental and/or substance use disorders. You can find them on the web at https://www.samhsa.gov/find-help/national-helpline

ONE LAST THING

One last thing before we move on to Perspective #2. We started this segment with my question, "What do I do if I recognize myself as one of the characters in the Addiction Monologues?" And my answer was to seek help.

The word "seek" is a verb - meaning it's an action we take. We attempt to find something - help. We attempt or **desire** to obtain something - help. We ask for something from someone - help.

If you want to heal from addition you must desire that healing and freedom above everything else. There is no such thing as failure in your pursuit of healing. You might make attempts, very heartfelt attempts, that don't produce your exact desired results you seek, but that isn't failure, that's part of your journey of healing and getting stronger. Thomas Edison made over one-thousand attempts at getting the lightbulb right. Edison's greatest strength was that he was brave enough (not afraid) to make an attempt. And when one of his attempts didn't light up the way he had hoped, he recognized it as a step in his journey to success, and he never stopped taking those necessary steps. Think about this every time you turn on a light. Now take a moment and check out, Ten Places to Start a Journey of Healing, in the Resource Section at the end of the book. Then come back and keep reading!

WE'RE NOT REALLY TALKING ABOUT THIS....
DON'T TELL....

The Secret Section

Disclaimer & Warning: *I'm going to talk about religion, spirituality, and I might mention a verse from the Bible. I do not consider these terms to be synonymous with one another. I'm confident that I may offend you at some point in this section, although it is not my intent. I'm apologizing in advance. Buckle your seatbelt.*

Addiction is a brain disease. That's public knowledge and is well documented by neuroscience.

But addiction is first and foremost a Spiritual disease. That's the secret no one wants to talk about. I believe addiction is a spiritual disease because it robs us of our purpose and significance as an image bearer of God. If you hold to a world view that does not allow for or contain a concept for God, that's fine and I'm not offended. I will modify the previous sentence to read - I believe addiction is a disease of purpose because it robs us of our purpose and significance as a human being.

Long before there was Functional Magnetic Resonance Imaging (fMRI) of the brain that could show how addiction highjacks or destroys normal brain function, the Apostle James wrote about it. Let me paraphrase what James wrote in chapter one, verses fourteen and fifteen of his letter in the New Testament of the Bible.

We are tempted by our own desires, which entice us and carry us away. These desires give birth to unhealthy habits or

patterns of living. When we allow these unhealthy (or morbid)
patterns to grow they result in death.

What are you tempted by? Personally I've never been tempted to eat Brussels sprouts. I hear they're good for me, but I've never been tempted to try them. Temptation is about pleasure, and or the reduction of my pain. It's all about feeling better. I can't imagine Brussels sprouts generating any form of pleasure or making me feel better. Neurologically speaking, Brussels sprouts do not produce a dopamine release. Hence, no temptation.

What do you desire? I desire a lot of things! The first thing that came to my mind wasn't world peace, but it probably should have been. Generally I desire things that would make my life easier, more fun, or more interesting (entertaining). When I'm in a lot of physical or emotional pain, I desire the pain to go away. I think it would be safe to say most people have that same desire.

If I'm experiencing significant physical or emotional pain, or soul crushing shame, my desire would be to get relief, and I would consider (be tempted by) almost anything that might promise that relief. The problem with many of our "less than healthy" behaviors is that most of them are addicting. They may not rise to the devastation caused by some street drugs, but they take you in the wrong direction.

The idea or concept of addiction is found in the last sentence of my paraphrase of James. When we allow these unhealthy (or morbid) patterns to grow, they result in death. First point - the habits grow. Especially if they make us "feel" better. Insert neuroscience: Better = dopamine release in the brain. Second point - unhealthy habits and morbidity. Unhealthy patterns of living decrease the quality of our physical, emotional and spiritual health. When we travel in a direction of decreasing quality of life, we eventually end up dead - spiritually, emotionally, and ultimately physically.

James nailed it. We desire our pain to go away. We are tempted and enticed by something that promises to do so. We engage that something. It grows in two ways; it gains more control over us and we lose control over it, and it moves us in a direction of diminishing health. The result is that we experience emotional, spiritual, and sometimes physical death, depending upon the activity or substance.

This process strips us of our created purpose and significance. But what starts the process in the first place? We all experience a lot of different pain in life. What is the source of the original pain? I believe it starts at the core of what addiction takes from us, purpose and significance. Lacking purpose and significance is a painful place to be, and the cycle (desire, temptation, enticement, use, growth of the habit, more negative consequences) spirals.

My journey with addiction and those suffering from it, has allowed me the sacred privilege of gaining unfiltered, raw access into the lives of many individuals. A lot of the words and phrases that have been spoken in my presence had never been uttered out loud for anyone else to hear. One such encounter was with a man I'll call Steve. He was forty when I met him, handsome and physically fit, the kind of man you would see on the cover of GQ or Men's Health magazine. Steve shared that he was a college graduate who had a very nice home, a beautiful wife, and two handsome sons. He had a high six-figure income, no debt, and all the expensive toys you could image that an income like that could buy. As he sat in my office, in his $1,000 suit, sharing these details about himself, he was in tears. As he finished telling me his story, he had only one question for me. "If I have all of this, why am I so f***ing miserable?"

Purpose and significance. Steve didn't understand either of these, and on top of that, he held a core belief that he "wasn't good enough." Everyone of us has both purpose and significance, but most of us don't know what they are, where they come from, or why we have them. Without a knowledge of our purpose and significance we will always be working hard at fending off the pain and never finding out. Addiction is standing by ready and more than willing to help us with that task of fending off the pain.

Addiction is a spiritual disease that robs us of our purpose and significance as an image bearer of God. If you believe we are created in the image of God, then we are made not only to do good things, but great things. Addiction destroys our ability to do that. It robs us of our purpose and significance as a human being. It is a disease of belief, *a belief in what is false. The belief that I don't matter, that I'm not good enough, and that no matter how hard I try, I never will be. One word captures all of this - shame.*

When this one false core belief is NOT successfully addressed and corrected, a person will not experience sustained healing from addiction. They may find temporary reprieve, sometimes lasting years or even decades, but addiction will find its way, its path, through substance or behavior, back into the person's life to "help" them relieve the emotional soul-ripping pain of not being enough.

Let me be clear, I'm not saying you should go find a church or religion in order to get well. Religion or church - I'm not assuming they are the same thing - can be helpful for you discovering and finding your purpose and the significance of your life. However, they can also be a vehicle that takes you to very dark places. Spiritual abuse is the fertile ground needed to cultivate an addictive behavior. Addiction rates for people that attend church are roughly the same as those who do not attend. What is needed is a spiritual awakening combined with a spiritual healing.

The Wound

Ultimately, the healing of addiction is about healing a spiritual wound. Some believe we are born with this wound, others would say we acquire it in early childhood. The wound is a false, lie-based belief about ourselves. The false belief is simple yet powerful. It is the belief that I don't matter, that I'm not good enough, and that no matter how hard I try, I never will be. The false belief is formed when our childhood developmental skills that are not capable of defending us in our thoughts. The belief is either formed by us, or given to us. Either way, once we have agreed to it, we begin to personalize it with every similar or reenforcing experience.

Prior to the age of ten, our brains are operating in a subconscious mode. In this mode, we can only accept ideas that are presented to us. That is why there is very little resistance to the ideas of Santa Claus, the Tooth Fairy, or the monster that we are told lives under our bed. It is only after the age of ten that our brain waves move to a higher frequency and we develop conscious thought. With conscious thought, we acquire the ability to reject thoughts and ideas. This is when we begin to challenge the idea of Santa Claus and the Tooth Fairy. However, when an early belief has been linked with a fear, such as the monster under our bed, it is much harder to adjust that false belief.

Healing

Healing from addiction is an inside job. We have a brain. We have a body. Individuals with a Western worldview usually talk about each of these as if they are separate from the other. What we struggle to understand is how our brain and body come together to form what we call our mind. Our beliefs about ourselves do not simply reside in our brain, they reside in our mind. Our mind is the unique and sometimes hard to describe confluence of our brain and our body. Listen carefully to what I'm about to say. We experience wounds from addiction in both our brain and in our body. But the wound that produces addiction resides in our mind.

Depending upon your philosophical or spiritual perspective, some might say this wound resides in our soul. Whether we identify the location of the wound to be in our mind or in our soul doesn't matter for this discussion. The point I am making is that it is a very deep wound.

Deep wounds take time to uncover. We often sense something is there, something is wrong, but we can't find words to describe it. We usually describe it by saying, I just don't feel right. That feeling is anchored in a belief. It is the belief that produces the feeling. We must understand that we don't change feelings, we change beliefs. Once a belief is changed, the feelings change.

I've known individuals with thirty years of abstinence and sobriety. Their body had completely recovered/healed from the adverse physical conditions resulting from their substance addiction. Their brain had also rebalanced and healed and their neurotransmitter chemicals that had been disrupted were now functioning as they should. But they relapsed, after thirty years. The "body" was healed and the "brain" was healed, but the core beliefs that resided in their mind were not healed.

Complete healing from addiction requires soul/mind repair. While addiction robs us of purpose and significance, it is the false belief that I don't matter, that I don't have a purpose or significance that allows addiction to form in the first place. Addiction is birthed when we don't believe and know that we have purpose and significance. If we really want to prevent addiction in any form, we need to help people discover and know their purpose and significance.

Healing and Daily Practice

Healing comes through daily physical, emotional, social, and spiritual practices. Get a picture in your mind of a wooden stool with four legs, each leg is connected to the others by spindles. Imagine yourself standing on top of this stool. You would want four, solid and sturdy legs on the stool to support you. You would want them all to be the same length firmly fastened together. Each leg of the stool represents one of these areas of daily practice, the physical, emotional, social, and spiritual aspects of your life. I'm very intentional about my use of the word practice rather than the word activity. Practice is about engaging in a behavior for a specific outcome. In this case, our desired outcome is healing that leads to a healthy and purpose oriented lifestyle.

Physical

At this moment how do you feel physically? Are you hungry? Are you warm? Cold? Did you get enough sleep last night? Should you be sleeping right now? Do you have any physical pain in your body? *What will you do* today to nurture your physical condition, and improve how you feel physically?

Emotional

What are you feeling emotionally right now? Content? Anxious? Fulfilled? Fearful? What has been your emotional theme for the past twenty-four hours? What will you do today to reduce your experience of fear or lower your anxiety? *What will you do* today to nurture

120

feelings of contentment and peace? What beliefs about yourself do you need to alter to improve what you are feeling emotionally?

Social Connection

Who have you connected with today? Do you have cheerleaders and supporters in your social circle? Or detractors and naysayers? Do your friends build you up and encourage you to grow? Does the social media sites you visit depress you or inspire you? _What will you do_ today to connect socially in a meaningful and healthier way? Will you be encouraged or will you be the encourager? Or both? Just a few hours ago, I received a voicemail from a friend who happened to be in recovery from an addiction. He prayed over me in my voicemail and finished his message with words of encouragement. He made me smile, and I wanted to be more like him. He also made me think about who I might need to reach out to and do the same. My connection with this friend made me a healthier person.

Spiritual (Purpose)

Why are you here on the planet? Do you know? Do you have a sense of purpose? Do you have a connection with something or someone greater than yourself? You have many talents and abilities. There is not another living creature in the universe exactly like you - you are a one of a kind masterpiece! We cannot move through time and space without making an impact. What impact will you make today? What will you do today to help yourself better understand your purpose? _What will you do_ today to nurture your awareness of God and your purpose?

What will you do? That phrase is underlined in each of the preceding paragraphs. A young mother of two small children helped me understand the importance to this question. I met her in an intensive outpatient substance abuse treatment group I was facilitating. Her drug of choice was prescription opiates - even though she didn't have a prescription. She was about four weeks into the treatment program when she relapsed and overdosed. She was at her house with her two

121

young children when it happened. Her husband found her on the back deck of their home unconscious and unresponsive. She was transported to the hospital by the paramedics and spent two days in ICU and was discharged the next day. She was back at the treatment group two days later recounting what had happened to her. As she told her story of overdosing she frequently inserted the phrase "I'll never do that again" and then continue with her story. After about the fifth or sixth time of hearing the phrase "I'll never do that again," I interrupted her story. I wasn't sure who she was trying to convince more of what she wasn't going to do, those of us in the group, or herself. And then, with respect and empathy, I told her I didn't care about what she <u>wasn't</u> going to do, I was more interested in what she <u>was</u> going to do.

As humans we often focus on what we don't want to do without really thinking about what we are going to do. Planning to not do something is not a plan of action, it is a plan of non-action. The real question that must be asked and answered is, what am I going to do?

In these daily practices, we not only heal, we also discover wounds we may not have been aware of that need healing. As we discover them, we need to bring them into the light, clean them, dress them, and allow the healing process to begin and take its course. Sometime that might require seeking help with the healing process from a trained professional. Treatment is not about fixing, it's about healing.

As you think about what you will do in each of the four daily practice areas, begin making a list of options that would work for you in each area. Either on a sheet of paper, in your phone, or on your computer, create a place to write down and store your ideas for each area.

Physical - Emotional - Social Connection - Spiritual

What moves an activity into the realm of practice is the intentionality of purpose in the activity. Take reading for example. Reading could be a possible activity to help us grow in the emotional or spiritual practice areas. Many people read the Big Book, the Twelve Steps, the Bible, or The Four Agreements. Very few people read them with the intentional purpose of life transformation. The pattern we usually fall into is we read something, and then we check the box, "read something today" and wait for something magical to happen. I remember a friend of mine after reading the Four Agreements for the first time coming back to me and saying, "If I could DO the stuff in this book it would completely transform my life!" She recognized there was a big difference between simply <u>reading about</u> the ideas presented and doing or <u>living out</u> the ideas. Reading about it is not living out. For a deeper dive into intentionality in each of the practice areas see Intentionality - Live it Out! in the Resource Section at the end of the book. While you are back there, also check out Twenty-Five Daily Practice Ideas.

Beginning the process of starting or enhancing your journey of healing is relatively simple - but not necessarily easy. Every day you must find the courage to do at least ONE thing that would fall into one of the practice areas. Within the next seven days, work up to doing ONE thing in EACH of the practice areas everyday. The key is to not simply check off a box like a "to do" list. This is so much more than doing! This is about BECOMING. Through the combination of your daily intentional effort in all four practice areas, you will become more of what your are seeking. You will begin to restore balance in life. As you do that, you will position yourself to discover and become more aware of your purpose and significance.

There is so much more that can be said about this journey of healing. It is an inside job - meaning only you can do it for yourself, but it's done with the support and love of others, and sometimes with well-trained therapists or coaches. So, if you are reading this as a "Perspective #1" person, I want to encourage you to get started AND ask for help. If you are a "Perspective #2" person and you're not already living a life that embraces these four daily practice areas, I want to encourage you to start as well. I want the Perspective #2 people to get started because this practice will enhance the quality of your life, provide some protection against addiction, and it will allow you to model a heathy, balanced lifestyle for your friend or family member that may be struggling. It will provide a framework for each of you to join and support each other. Begin your healing.

End of The Secret Section

Disclaimer & Warning: *My intent was not to offend, but at times that cannot be avoided. I know I apologized in advance of this section, but I'm not really sorry* 😬 *. Some topics are just hard to talk about and my hope was to present this section with empathy, respect, and sensitivity to a multiple of world views. Hopefully that wasn't too painful. The seatbelt sign has been turned off and you are free to go refill your coffee.*

(Remember - Don't tell anyone about this part!)

PERSPECTIVE #2
I RECOGNIZE SOMEONE ELSE IN THE ADDICTION MONOLOGUES

What do I do if I recognize a friend or family member as one of the characters in the Addiction Monologues? You will need to do several things, simultaneously. You offer to help them, while at the same time learning to interact with them in a way that doesn't fuel their struggle. I'm going to try and address both of these simultaneously just like I asked you to do. Before we jump into how you do that, I need to say one thing. Breathe. Deep breaths, several of them, do that now.

SELF-CARE

"My daughter either needs to get well...or she needs to die....because we can't do this any longer." Those were the very honest words spoken in a family group by an exhausted father. He was the father of the young woman I modeled the character of Julie after in the monologue. He was brave enough to say what everyone else in the room was thinking and feeling. After he said it he broke down and started sobbing wanting to know what they had done wrong.

If we don't wrestle with the storyline of the monologue, the experience of reading it will be of little value. I want you to know that the characters presented in the monologue are actual people. I did change their names, age, race, and gender, except for the getting pregnant storyline. While it is a work of fiction, it really isn't fiction. The events and details were not loosely based upon someone's life story - every event and detail actually happened to someone just like you or me. What the monologue fails to portray is the pain of all the family members and friends who appear as backstory of the monologue. The real-life mother of the character of Peter sat in my office and told me about watching her son eat the Lyrica out of her toilet. It's all real.

Living in the world of addiction is hard, ugly, heart wrenching, and exhausting. If you've lived in or near this world you probably have a few more descriptors to add to the list. When we are physically, emotionally, and spiritually exhausted, it's hard to help ourselves, let alone another person. Self-care is a must! It is about healing and being healthy. It is also about modeling healthy practices for your friend or family member. You just read about self-care in the Secret Section under the subheading, Healing and Daily Practice. As a Perspective #2 person, you also need these daily practices in your life. I want to encourage you to get started with them and look at both Intentionality - Live it Out! and Twenty-Five Daily Practice Ideas in the Resource Section at the end of the book. Your intentional self care will help your loved one or friend in their journey of healing. They will have a stronger person by their side who can join with them in this journey of getting well.

RESPONDING TO AN "ASK FOR HELP"

Remember Addiction's strategy from the monologue?

"It's a standard part of my strategy to isolate my prey. The isolation intensifies the loneliness and helps to slowly build the pain. It's an easy strategy with humans because you actually think it helps – you reason that if you don't have to talk about "it" or have to explain "it" then, "it" will be less painful. Most often you work with me in this strategy by humiliating your fellow humans. It all works so well."

I mean this with all sincerity, addiction doesn't need any help, especially from you. Your loved one needs your help and they are asking you for it. Help your loved one, don't help Addiction. Remember Karen in the monologues? She wanted to share her struggle with her parents, but they didn't have time to listen. Perspective #2 people, please have time and listen without judgment or shame.

Several pages ago I told your loved one or friend that, "There will be a reaction when you ask for help." What would your reaction be if someone you knew, who trusted you, shared their ugly secret with you in hopes that you would help them? Please read that question again. I want you to really think through how you would act or react if someone you knew revealed their struggle with addiction and asked for help. We are talking about the difference between acting and reacting. My first suggestion to you, if it would feel appropriate, would be to give them a big hug, hold it for at least twenty-thirty seconds, and say nothing. Holding a hug for at least twenty-thirty seconds will cause our brain to release the neurotransmitter/peptide hormone oxytocin. This will happen in both of you. Oxytocin produces a feeling of connection and bonding. Part of its purpose is to create a sense of safety. And feeling safe would be a high priority need for both of you in this situation.

How you respond, act or react, to someone coming to you with their secret struggle is so very important and critical to what happens next. The person in front of you, your loved one or friend, has been experiencing the soul crushing weight of shame and guilt that comes with addiction. Every thought in their mind and feeling in their body screams, "Don't do it! Don't let them know! They won't understand, they'll think you're weak and disgusting! Don't talk to them about it!" When in reality, asking for help is one of the bravest most courageous things they could do. Never shame a person that is asking for help. Honor their courage and bravery with respect and kindness.

"Shame - The intensely painful feeling or experience of believing that we are flawed and therefore unworthy of love and belonging – something we've experienced, done, or failed to do makes us unworthy of connection." - Brené Brown

Understanding Shame - We often use the words guilt and shame interchangeably. They are not. Guilt is the sense or feeling I experience after I have DONE something wrong. Shame is the sense or feeling that I AM wrong, no matter what I do. Shame is more than an emotion or feeling, it is a belief that becomes our identity. And shame is toxic. You don't need to add any, addiction provides a more than adequate supply. Be sure to take a look at **Shame: The approach that keeps producing exactly what you don't want,** in the resource session.

  If you want to help a Perspective #1 person, someone who is caught in addiction, you will have to navigate through their shame. Shame is painful. It's a dull pain when you don't touch it, it's a sharp soul-piercing pain when you do touch it. So we don't want to touch it. Our approach needs to be one of an unconditional, positive regard for our loved one or friend. An unconditional, positive regard means respecting people and honoring them as fellow human beings, especially when they are reaching out to us for help with addiction.

After you get done with that hug to help release some oxytocin into the room, you will want to take action. Don't ask questions like "How did this happen?" or "Why didn't you come to me sooner?" or "What were you thinking?" All of which could trigger shame and won't add any value to the next task. The next thing on the to-do list is to begin movement towards healing. While we're on the topic of things to not say or ask, don't say, "Let's get you into treatment." Treatment is a very scary word for someone suffering with addiction. It's like saying to someone just diagnosed with cancer "Let's get you into chemotherapy!" Stick with words like help and healing.

The action you take next will depend upon the condition of your friend or loved one. If you have any concerns about their physical health, such as apparent symptoms of withdrawals, I strongly urge you to take them to an ER or Urgent Care to be checked out and medically cleared. If your loved one is alcohol dependent showing signs of withdrawal with a fever or seizures, there is no question, take them somewhere to get medical care or call 911. The mortality rate from severe alcohol withdrawal and delirium tremens (DT) has been as high as 25% in some studies.

If your loved one or friend is not in immediate medical danger, you will want to begin looking at different paths to connect with resources. I've included the guide Ten Places to Start a Journey of Healing in the Resource Section to help you with identifying the next steps the two of you will take together. I want to encourage you to walk WITH your friend or loved one through this journey. Remember the woman I mentioned earlier who came to the appointment with her co-worker? Be that person! The person that says to their friend "I'm with you and will be there for you."

OFFERING HELP

Where do we begin? Let's begin with the elephant in the room. It's not pink like an exaggerated cartoon caricature, and it's not smiling. It's big, smelly, weighs over twelve thousand pounds, leaves messes commensurate with its size, and you often feel like it's sitting on your chest.

Offering help can be a hard step to take. Offering help is an act of courage. If your timing isn't just right, you will experience rejection. Don't take it personally. I know that is much easier said than done. Hopefully by now you're beginning to grasp the emotional, spiritual, and neuroscience complexity of addiction. It is that complexity we must navigate as we offer help. What we offer must match the stage of change our loved one or friend happens to be in at the moment, and that frequently changes moment by moment.

THE STAGES OF CHANGE

Precontemplation
Contemplation
Preparation
Action
Maintenance

The "stages of change" are five basic stages we all go through when attempting to change one of our behavioral patterns. The first stage is precontemplation, meaning we're not thinking about change at all. It's simply not on our radar. The second stage, contemplation, means exactly that, I've started to THINK about making a change, but physically I'm still sitting on the couch and there is no action taking place. We start to see physical movement in the preparation stage. We might see quite a bit of activity in this stage and we have to be careful not to confuse that preparation activity with action. The action stage is where the real healing work takes place, usually in professional treatment. The final stage is the maintenance stage where we are able to maintain our new behavioral habit without relapsing back into our previous pattern.

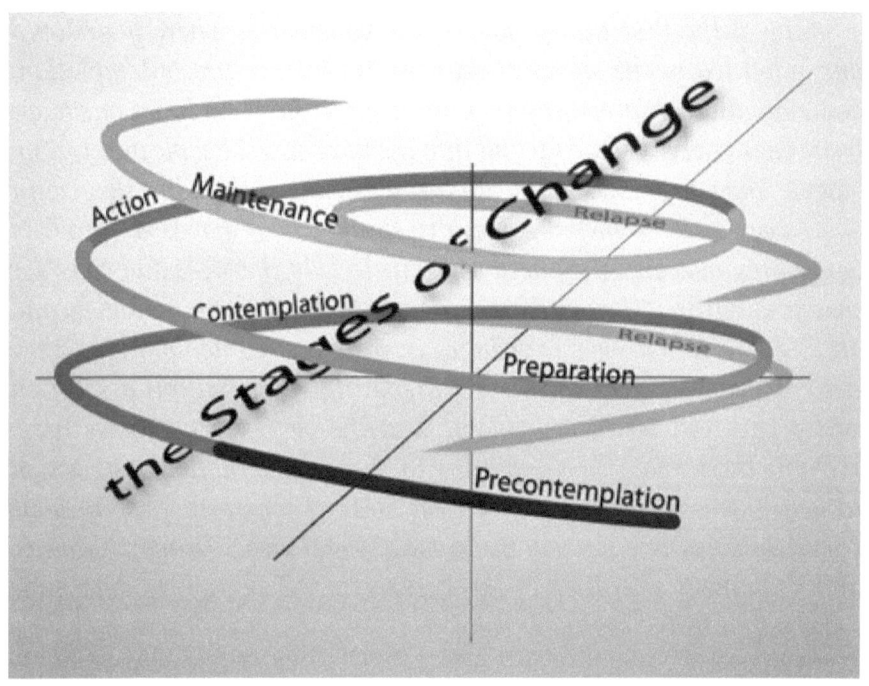

Our journey through these stages is more like a spiral than a straight line. Relapse is not just about returning to a behavior, it's about returning to a way of thinking. One moment I'm thinking about (Contemplation) going to the gym to exercise, and the next moment I've relapsed back into precontemplation and I'm lying on the couch eating ice cream. One moment your loved one can be looking at treatment facilities on the internet with you and talking about which one looks like a good fit for them, and the next day they're fine and don't need to go. Some research indicates that 40% of individuals with addictions related to substances are in precontemplation, another 40% are in contemplation, and only 20% are in preparation.

Don't be discouraged by those figures. Your loved one or friend is blessed to have YOU in their life. You've read the Monologue and you now know some of "Addiction's secrets." With that knowledge you are now in a better place to help your loved one or friend. You're making a courageous decision to offer help and they are fortunate to have you on their side. Be patient with yourself and the process.

One of the first things you should consider is where your loved one is located in the stages of change. Are they in precontemplation, contemplation, or preparation? Our goal is to help our loved one move from their current stage up and into the next stage. People don't jump stages. They might move quickly through some of them but they don't skip them. If someone doesn't think they have a problem (precontemplation), they need someone to help them see and consider that possibility. If they already recognize they may have a problem and are needing to make some changes in their life (contemplation), they need someone to help them start preparing (preparation) a solution and a path out of their problem. And the biggest step comes next. Helping them move from preparing to change to actually taking action to help them get well. For practical ideas of where to go with your friend or loved one, review the areas of Employers, Support Groups, and Treatment Facilities in the Perspective #1 section to determine what might be the best next step.

OFFERING HELP WITH L. O. V. E.

A simple way to organize your offer of help is with the acronym - LOVE.

  L – Let them know you love them and why.
  O – Offer examples of why you're concerned.
  V – Validate the difficulty of their situation and
    struggle.
  E – Encourage them to accept your offer to walk with
    them and get the help they need.

  I recommend writing out a brief narrative based upon this acronym. You will want to at least jot down some notes for yourself to help you stay on track with what you want to say. You don't need to write a novel, just three-four sentences for each letter section. If you were offering help to a friend or co-worker you would adapt what you say to the level of the relationship and talk about caring for them versus what you love about them. I've included some short narrative examples in the More Resources section at the end of the book to help you out with this.

SOME FINAL THOUGHTS

"Insanity is doing the same thing over and over again and expecting different results." Attributed to Albert Einstein

If we want a different outcome regarding addiction, we need to think differently. In order to think differently we need to look at addiction from as many different (new) perspectives as possible. We need to be creative in our approach. We need to look through as many different lenses as possible, and maybe even create some new ones. My hope is that the Addiction Monologues has helped you to see a different perspective. Whether you identify with perspectives #1 or #2, I want to encourage you and ask you to do at least one or more of the following:

Ask for help. I know I've encouraged and suggested several times that you ask for help. I'm reminded of the December 1st reading of AA's Daily Reflections book. It talks about how the Twelve Steps is a "suggested" plan for recovery. The passage goes on to say when a paratrooper jumps out of an airplane it's "suggested" that they pull their ripcord. Personally I have skydived, and I highly recommend/suggest pulling the ripcord. Ask for help, it's a suggestion, but your life really does depend upon it.

Accept any help that is offered to you, then build upon it.

Give this book to someone else. Addiction wants us to shut up and stop talking about this ugly topic. Keep the discussion going! Be as unconventional as you have to be to save a life, whether it's yours or someone else.

**** MORE RESOURCES ****

SHAME
~ THE APPROACH THAT KEEPS PRODUCING EXACTLY WHAT YOU DON'T WANT

We all know what shame feels like. It's a powerful motivating force. Take a moment, reflect, think of a time in your life when feeling shame moved you to take a positive action or step in your life. Have you thought of one? Keep trying.....Still thinking? You're probably having a hard time finding a memory where the voice of shame came through in your mind and said, "Yes! You can do this! Stand up! Speak up! Take the leap!" Instead you probably remember something more like this - "What the hell are you doing! SIT DOWN! Don't look, don't make eye contact. Find the door, where's the door, we need to get out of here, this was a terrible idea!"

The primary action we take when feeling shame is to hide or to want to get away from the source that is triggering our shame. Everyone knows that shame has never motivated them to move in a positive direction. So why do we think it will work on someone else? The problem is with our logic. We think we can use shame to get someone to stop engaging in a bad or unhealthy behavior. Google the current prison population if you're wondering how well this logic works.

Shame, as Brené Brown describes it is, the intensely painful feeling or experience of believing that we are flawed and therefore unworthy of love and belonging – something we've experienced, done, or failed to do makes us unworthy of connection. Shame is several things all at the same time. It is a slow acting toxin that causes us to live an emotionally painful existence that ultimately leads to emotional/mental and physical illness. It is a slow acting poison that ultimately kills us. At the same time, however, it can also be like a shot of adrenaline - think four shots of expresso - that causes our heart to start beating out of our chest and fuels an overwhelming desire to do

138

whatever it takes to escape from whoever is poking our shame-based beliefs.

The opposite of shame is an unconditional, positive regard. We need to be sure we understand what this phrase means. The term "unconditional" refers to the positive regard, or dignity, we offer someone. Unconditional does NOT refer to condoning bad, threatening, or unhealthy behavior or actions by someone. We respect the dignity of the person without condoning or allowing their actions to go on without consequence. But the consequence of a bad choice cannot be shaming. It is possible to show and offer someone positive regard (dignity and human respect) unconditionally, and still have and maintain appropriate boundaries.

Let's call it the "Law of Shame." The use of shaming will never produce long-term positive (healthy) behavioral change. In fact, if you use shame as an approach to stop or change someones behavior, it will only be a matter of time before they will produce the exact same behavior you were trying to deter or extinguish. Shame begets shame, which then fuels behaviors people think will take away their pain. But the behaviors themselves don't take the pain away. The only real solution to the pain caused by shame or trauma is healing. Shame is an approach that will keep producing exactly what you don't want.

INTENTIONALITY ~ LIVE IT OUT!

"I'm just going through the motions." If we haven't said it out loud, we've thought it in our head at some point. We go through the motions, not really present, in order to check a box or check something off the list. I've worked with many people who have said they've "done" the Twelve Steps, or they've "done" treatment, or they've "read" that particular book, yet they don't experience lasting healing and behavioral change. There are many reasons some people struggle more than others in the healing process. I believe one of the reasons we struggle with the change process is that we don't live into the process. It doesn't matter which change process we're attempting to follow (AA, NA, CR, SMART, The 4 Agreements) simply doing it will not be enough, we have to live out the process.

Doing something with intention means we do it with purpose. Without intentionality there is no transformation. Our purpose must be to experience transformation. For this to take place we must be fully present in the moment and in the activity, whatever that happens to be. I'm not saying this is easy or simple. We're fighting against our cultural programing that tells us to coast whenever we can. Being mindful takes a level of effort most of us have never been taught to master.

Let's start with being present in the moment. The way we engage a moment in the physical world is through our senses. Just before I sat down to work on this section of the book, I was at a coaching appointment at an automotive shop. The shop had seven bays for working on vehicles. Each bay was occupied with a vehicle undergoing some form of maintenance. Imagine for a moment what the shop smelled like. Your mind might be bringing up a mixture of gasoline and exhaust with some oil and maybe the smell of rubber tires. Imagine for a moment what sounds were coming from the shop. Here's a twist. I arrived just after lunch time, and they had been grilling burgers and hotdogs. Smell it? Taste it?

Your mind just brought you into the moment I shared with you. You experienced it at a different level because I prompted you to engage your sense of smell, hearing, and taste. Even though you weren't there, you now have some level of shared awareness with me in the experience. Engaging our senses will help us to be present in the moment. It is the use of our physical senses that make us aware.

In a different, but similar fashion, we also can sense our emotions. When I walked into that auto shop I could tune into my physical senses and tell you if it was warm, cold, or just right, what it smelled like and what it sounded like. But what was I feeling? Was I feeling excitement over the opportunity to connect with my clients? Or some anxiety over what they might share with me and whether I would be able to effectively coach them? Or was I feeling excitement or anxiety over something that had happened early in the day? Or were my emotions connected to what I was anticipating later in the evening? Was I emotionally (mentally) present in the room?

We must be both physically and emotionally present in the moment to fully live out the moment with intention. Now let's poke at intention. Intention is a mental state that reflects a level of commitment to something. I like the way Vocabulary.com describes it: If you are intent on doing something, you are determined to get it done. If you have an intent, you have a motive or purpose.

Do I know the purpose of my actions? Let's be honest with ourselves. If I internally state my purpose and intent to "go through the motions," I'm stating that my purpose and intent is not to be transformed, but rather to exert the least amount of physical, mental, and emotional energy as possible. Which begs the question, why then am I going through the motions? Just save yourself some time and do something else.

This is where it gets subconsciously more complicated. We all have beliefs deep within us that we formed at a young age that sound something like "I'm not good enough, smart enough, or something else enough." Or we phrase it in the other direction "I'm too bad, too dumb, or too slow." Either way, we have created a lid for ourselves.

We create a limiting belief based upon not having enough of a good quality or having too much of a bad quality that internally (subconsciously) stops us from being able to move forward with our intention to grow, change, improve, or heal. And we don't have just one. We usually have a large interconnected network of limiting beliefs. When we become aware of one of them, we have to reject it, delete it, and replace it. This is the process of awareness. It is not an event, it is a lifestyle. It is a living skill.

As we increase in our awareness of what we believe about ourselves and release our limiting beliefs, we develop a lifestyle of intentionally. We live out our life with the intent to grow, to heal, to become healthier. Growing and healing becomes our intent, it becomes our purpose.

TEN PLACES
TO START A JOURNEY OF HEALING

Here are ten possible places to start a journey of healing. They are not listed in order of significance or priority. They are simply possible starting points for you to consider as you explore options. If you try one of these options and it fails to deliver the support you need, don't stop, pick another and keep trying until you get connected with the resources that are helpful for you.

Your local ER or Urgent Care - *If you are feeling emotionally or physically desperate, like you can't go on and don't want or care if you make it into tomorrow, this is the place to start. Ask someone to take you, contact Uber, or call 911 to get there. The staff at the ER or Urgent Care will make sure you're safe, and they will also help you get connected with the resources you need to continue your journey.*

Your Primary Care Physician - *If you have a visit coming up soon with your doctor they are the perfect person to ask about getting the help you need. Either the doctor or a member of their staff should be able to help you with the next steps, and provide you with the support you need and the connections for further ongoing support.*

Google - Or the search engine of your choice - *An internet search can help you locate and narrow down your search for the remaining locations on this list. It can also help you with specifics on hours of operation, meeting times, program and staff descriptions, accreditations, downloadable forms and other useful information. When using a search engine always explore three-four of the search results and always look to see if "Ad" appears before the web address in the result. The "Ad" means someone has paid money to be put at the top of the list and they may not be exactly what you're looking for.*

SAMHSA's National Helpline – 1-800-662-HELP(4357) - *Substance Abuse and Mental Health Services Administration - SAMHSA's National Helpline is a free, confidential, 24/7, 365-day-a-year treatment referral and information service in English and Spanish. You can also find it at* https://www.samhsa.gov/find-help/national-helpline.

Local Support Groups - *There are a variety of support groups that can serve as first steps in your journey of healing. If you search on any of these program names you should find options close to your location. Many of them also operate online programs that you can connect with immediately.*

- *Alcoholics Anonymous*
- *Al Anon*
- *Celebrate Recovery*
- *Narcotics Anonymous*
- *SMART Recovery*

Employee Assistance Program (EAP) Program - *Your place of employment may offer an Employee Assistance Program. Check with your Human Resource Department or supervisor for contact information. You might be able to connect with them over the phone or go in person. They usually provide up to three visits at no cost and they can help you confidentially connect with the specific resources that would best fit your needs.*

Individual Private Practice Therapist or Counselor - *If you make a web search for "Therapists near me" you will no doubt get a long list of counseling connecting sites. Many of them will be for online connection and not in person. If you want to start your journey with a therapist or counselor, I would recommend meeting with someone in person. I would recommend* https://www.psychologytoday.com/us/therapists *for locating a therapist in your area. This site offers several screening filters and a* lot of useful information. Be sure to look for addiction treatment experience and certifications such as the CAADC.

A Treatment Facility - *Just to be clear, connecting with a treatment facility doesn't necessarily mean going away for twenty-eight days. There are all types of treatment facilities and all offer a range of services and treatment levels which could include, outpatient care, intensive- outpatient care, partial hospitalization, and inpatient care. A good treatment program will match the level of care to the needs of the individual. You can usually start the screening process with a phone call. They will have a lot of questions for you, answer honestly, it's confidential. No one can effectively help you if they don't have an accurate picture. Remember to ask your own questions as well, and take notes or have someone else take notes:*

- *Is the treatment facility accredited?*
- *Is the facility licensed by the state?*
- *What is the level of training for your staff? Do you have recovery coaches?*
- *Are you affiliated with any religious organizations, faiths, or church?*
- *Do you provide both detoxification services and treatment services?*
- *What kind of after-care support do you offer or provide?*

You can make a web search for treatment facilities in your area or you could use the SAMHSA's website treatment locator or helpline mentioned earlier.

Recovery Coach - *A recovery coach is a person who is trained, and sometimes licensed, to assist people in their recovery and healing journey. They have been there - in the monologue - and are now on the other side. They can be especially helpful in supporting you and connecting you with the resources you might need on your journey. If you are feeling unsure about this whole process, you might try* connecting over a coffee with a recovery coach in your area just to hear their perspective and maybe give you some ideas. One way to locate a recovery coach would be to call some of your local treatment providers, and inquire if they have a coach on their staff that you could speak with.

Church or Place of Worship - *It is not uncommon for churches or other places of worship to furnishing space for support groups for their meetings. Even if you are not attending that church, or any church for that matter, you can look on the church website and usually find out if they host or provide recovery-based programming. They will usually list a contact person or meeting times. Some churches also offer confidential, low cost counseling services similar to the EAP program mentioned earlier. You could use this service to help connect you with additional resources.*

These are suggestions. Be creative, use more than one. Be committed and intentional in finding and connecting with the help you need.

TWENTY-FIVE DAILY PRACTICE IDEAS

Every one of these ideas come from people I've worked with over the years. Be creative. You can combine ideas as well. You might do some of these things daily, weekly, or just once a month. Think of the list as a menu you can choose from. The goal is to make sure that you are doing something that will have a positive refueling impact in one or more of the 4 impact areas:

Physical - Emotional - Social Connection - Spiritual

1. *Read a daily passage from a meditation or reflection book.* ** *Emotional and Spiritual impact*
2. *Do Yoga or Tai Chi individually.* ** *Physical and Emotional impact*
3. *Attend an AA, CR, or SMART meeting.* ** *Spiritual and Social impact*
4. *Spend at least five-seven minutes in focused breathing and mindfulness relaxation.* *** *Physical, Emotional, and Spiritual impact*
5. *Go for a walk by yourself.* ** *Physical and Emotional impact*
6. *Attend a Yoga or Tai Chi in a group class.* *** *Physical, Emotional, and Social impact*
7. *Spend time writing in a journal and reflecting on your thoughts.* ** *Emotional and Spiritual impact*
8. *Skip the junk food and eat a healthy meal.* ** *Physical and Emotional impact*
9. *Pray.* ** *Emotional and Spiritual impact*
10. *Join with a group of like-minded individuals for prayer.* ** *Emotional, Spiritual, and Social impact*

11. Read a self-improvement book. ** Emotional and Spiritual impact

12. Get a membership at a local gym (and go to it). *** Physical, Emotional, and Social impact

13. Listen to Bilateral Stimulation Music for at least seven-ten minutes during the day. Example: Bilateral Music - Bryan Cumming *** Physical, Emotional, and Spiritual impact

14. Find a quarter mile running track and walk four or more laps. Have a topic or thought focus for each lap. *** Physical, Emotional, and Spiritual impact

15. Do #14 with another person or small group. **** Physical, Emotional, Spiritual impact, and Social impact

16. Get out your camera and find something beautiful or interesting to take a picture of and try to find beauty every day. ** Emotional and Spiritual impact

17. Get a sketch book and draw in pencil or colored pencil - at least one doodle or sketch per day. ** Emotional and Spiritual impact

18. Get a plant and devote at least two-three minutes of attention and nurture to it daily, see if you can make it grow and flourish. ** Emotional and Spiritual impact

19. Watch at least one sunrise or sunset each week, or daily. *** Physical, Emotional, and Spiritual impact

20. Put a breathing app on your phone and use it daily. ** Physical and Emotional impact

21. Find an essential oil that has a unique smell that you enjoy and use it daily. ** Physical and Emotional impact

22. Hot bath with an essential oil. ** Physical and Emotional impact

23. Write a couple of sentences that reflect your purpose and read them daily. ** Emotional and Spiritual impact.

24. Paint something! It doesn't have to be fancy, keep it small and simple - the goal is to create. *** Physical, Emotional, and Spiritual impact.

25. *Text an affirmation or positive statement to a friend.* ***
    Emotional, Spiritual, and Social impact

L. O. V. E.

Here are a few bare bone examples of how to organize your thoughts using the L.O.V.E structure:

  L – Let them know that you love them and why you love them.

  O – Offer examples of why you are concerned.

  V – Validate the difficulty of their situation and struggle.

  E – Encourage them to accept your offer to walk with them and get the help they need.

<u>Example for a friend or coworker</u>:

"You know I care about you as a co-worker and fellow human being. It looks like life might be throwing a few things at you right now that you are struggling with. I know it can be tough, and I'm not even going to pretend I know what it's like to be in your situation. I just want to encourage you. It's okay to ask for help, and I'm here to help you if I can. Just let me know."

<u>Example for a loved one, family member, or very close friend</u>:

"I've been thinking about you. You know I love you. You have done so many things for me over the years and helped me out in so many different ways [you could give a specific example here]. I can see your struggling with the alcohol [example - last week at the restaurant you had way too many and ended up saying some things I know you regret]. I can't imagine how difficult the struggle might be or what it feels like for you. I do know there's a lot of help out there, and I want to encourage you to connect with some of it. I know of a few resources we could look into for help, and I'd be happy to go with you and check them out. In fact, I'd insist on going with you because I don't want you to do this alone. What do you say?"

ABOUT THE AUTHOR

Richard Campbell is a life coach, therapist, speaker, and author. As a former Intelligence Officer, he has trained over 1,000 Intelligence Officers in thinking and analytical skills for the United States Air Force. He has helped countless others improve their physical and emotional health and performance in life. As the founder of Living Well - Leading Well, he trains individuals and teams to become healthy, high performers in life, work, and business. In addition to a degree in Physical Science, he holds advanced degrees in Social Work and Political Science and has advanced certifications in trauma treatment and addiction treatment. His clients have included Fortune 500 executives, entrepreneurs, engineers, musicians, painters, martial artists, moms, dads, as well as college and high school students. He would love to encourage and inspire you! Follow him on Instagram at @livingwell.leadingwell

www.ingramcontent.com/pod-product-compliance
Lightning Source LLC
Chambersburg PA
CBHW021417210526
45463CB00001B/416